Table of Contents

REVIEWS

What a great read! In this book, Kate presents the facts on many childhood health concerns, from illness to diet/lifestyle. As a registered pediatric nurse, I enjoyed reading this well written manual full of practical advice and alternatives to Western medicine and health care. It was refreshing to read about childhood illness from the viewpoint of a well-studied mother (after all, who knows their child better?), with research based facts to back up the information given. I strongly recommend this book to all parents who want to save time, stress, money, and unnecessary trips to healthcare faciltities by being empowered to prevent and treat minor childhood illness.

Holly of Whole Sweet Home

A Practical Guide to Children's Health is a must have book for every family. Kate covers everything from nutrition and health to exercise and schooling options. I wish all my friends and family with children would buy this book. I am excited to have it as part of my collection. I will be referencing this book again and again.

Katie of Nourishing Simplicity

Every parent needs a tool like Kate Tietje's "Practical Guide to Children's Health" -- a quick guide to managing everyday child health problems. Scraped knee? Flip through the book and apply the wisdom. Ringworm? Try a few natural remedies before your doc prescribes a systemic anti-fungal. Kate will point you to some first line defense options. New parents and those new to real food eating will especially appreciate Kate's discussion of educating children about food and helping them learn healthy eating habits.

Amanda Rose, Ph.D., author *Rebuild from Depression: A Nutrient Guide*
http://www.Traditional-Foods.com

A Practical Guide to Children's Health

FOREWORD

As a pediatric and prenatal chiropractor, I get to see just about everything you can imagine when it comes to children's health. From ear infections to whooping cough to asthma to autism; you name it and I have probably seen it. The average childin this country will get multiple colds, flus, ear infections and any number of other illnesses per year. An astonishing 50% of kids are now afflicted with some form of chronic disease. Many doctors will try to reassure parents by telling them that they see this all the time and it is normal. In my opinion, this may be common but it is not normal.

When children get sick, the average parent will run to the medicine cabinet for a medication to suppress the symptoms. Others will rush to their pediatrician's office demanding a prescription for an antibiotic or some other drug. Most of the time, these well-intentioned doctors are only too happy to comply because their training dictates that they prescribe drugs to treat symptoms. I find that few parents are ever informed about the possible side-effects of these drugs and none are educated about the negative consequences associated with the suppression of these symptoms likely because the physicians themselves have never been taught the purpose, or dare I say benefits, of illness.

So why do kids get sick? In my experience, truly healthy kids rarely get sick and, when they do, it is often a short-lived experience that results in a stronger and more robust child. Sadly our modern food supply and eating habits are devoid of many of the essential nutrients kids require in order to maintain a healthy body and immune system. Added to that is an accumulation of toxins from exposure to genetically modified foods (GMOs), pesticides, vaccines, prescription drugs, chlorinated swimming pools, fluoridated water and a host of other insults. Over time, these deficiencies and toxicities build up and allow germs to take root in this weakened and diseased tissue. These germs reprodu ce and, in some cases, release toxins of their own resulting in clinical symptoms of illness. These symptoms, such as congestion, cough and the dreaded fever feared by parents and doctors alike, are merely an attempt by the body to mobilize its defenses and detoxify in order to restore the health of the child. It is a healing reaction. Suppression of these symptoms through synthetic pharmaceutical intervention inhibits the body's ability to detoxify, increases the toxic load and can ultimately result in more severe secondary complications. An illness can only overwhelm a child if the toxic build-up is extreme, the nutritional deficiencies are significant and the ability of the immune system to respond appropriately is impaired.

Not too long ago, a parent asked me if I could recommend a book that would help her address her children's health issues naturally at home. Nothing came to mind. I explained to her that what I knew had come from the research and experience I had acquired through my years in pediatric practice. Today I would have a different answer. "A Practical Guide To Children's Health" by Kate Tietje is an extremely comprehensive and well-researched resource for parents looking for natural alternatives to keep their children happy and healthy. This book will provide you with invaluable information whether you are a first-time parent or a veteran mom.

Readers are taken on a journey into a wide variety of children's health issues touching on everything from acute illness to chronic disease. She provides parents with a wide array of practical options for boosting kids' immunity naturally in order to prevent illness as well as treating common childhood illnesses at home. I can vouch for the effectiveness of many of these remedies having seen them provide great results in my practice and home over the years.

She provides an excellent in-depth discussion about the importance of nutrition and the many pitfalls parents face as they try to navigate the clever marketing and misinformation expounded by food companies and government health authorities. Readers also benefit from some affordable, healthy recipes that she uses in her home and guidance on how to get the whole family involved. I definitely learned some things that have been helpful in our home.

The book concludes with an investigation into common environmental insults that can affect a child's health. Parents will learn about everything from safe bedding to avoiding toxic personal care products. I can say, without hesitation, that her knowledge of these issues far surpasses that of most doctors. This book is definitely an asset to every parent and pediatric health-care provider. My hope is that it helps you to restore and retain your children's most precious asset...their health.

Dr. Tyson Perez, D.C., owner of West Coast Chiropractic in Carlsbad, CA

INTRODUCTION

INTRODUCTION

I'll be honest.

When my first baby came along, I knew nothing about health. I *thought* I did. I ate lots of salads and fruit and homemade soups while I was pregnant (canned fruits and store-bought salad dressing). I also ate lots of low-fat boxed meals and took OTC drugs to manage morning sickness. I didn't gain too much weight and I didn't have any complications. I breastfed. I took children's chewable vitamins. I was "healthy."

What a wake-up call it was a year after my daughter was born to realize that her frequent night waking, terrible eczema, constant diaper rash, and near-constant diarrhea weren't normal. Everyone told me not to worry about these things. "They're common. Many kids have these." That may be true, but it wasn't okay.

That started our journey to *real* health. As I've researched and read and had more babies, I've learned more and more about what produces a healthy baby and child, as well as how to "fix" one who was born when you didn't know any better. It's never too late to make changes, and you should never feel guilty for what you didn't know.

There are so many different areas to consider – food, medicine, clothing, personal care products, and even more!

Keep kids healthy isn't as hard as it looks, even if you didn't "start" right and are coming at it with older kids. I've done that too. It can be a rough transition but believe me, it's worth it.

Remember: I'm just a mom, like you. This book is based on what I've learned over the past 5 years or so of "being mom" to four children. It's not a substitute for medical advice and shouldn't be treated as such. If you're looking for another mom's advice and research, this is a great place to start! Please take any concerns or questions about particular remedies or nutritional needs (or anything else) to your child's pediatrician or another health professional. See my disclaimer for more!

If you're looking for a practical guide to keep your kids healthier, this is it. Come join me!

WHY I'M WRITING THIS BOOK

It took me a good three years to start researching what it took to keep my kids healthy and actually make sense of it all. There is so much conflicting information out there! I tried out different things on different kids, read different books, talked to different professionals, as I tried to navigate "the" right way to keep my kids healthy.

It can be seriously crazy-making. Think about it – eggs are good; eggs are bad. The flu causes autism – no, the flu *shot* does! How is a parent supposed to know what to believe with conflicting "studies" coming out almost daily?

Most parents just don't have the time or energy to do such research, and they want to rely on a few important resources. In many cases, pediatricians serve as this resource. There are some *excellent* pediatricians out there, but I've also heard some pretty terrible advice from a few. I definitely consult with mine over any important matter and I trust most of what he says, but I don't take his advice as the be-all, end-all. I know my kids the best, and he sees them for thirty minutes annually.

I'm hoping this book can serve as a resource for parents who don't know where to start their research, don't know how to make practical changes, and don't have hundreds of hours to spend figuring it out. The book is meant as a basic guide to keeping kids healthy through what they eat, the medicine they use for acute illnesses, and what's in their environment.

All of this is based on the knowledge that I've gathered through my hundreds of hours of research, reading many sources, talking to several professionals, and experimenting. It's, shall we say, "folk wisdom" of sorts. It contains over three hundred sources (so you can look directly at the studies for more information, if you like) and many of these are medical journals or other primary sources. It's not medical advice, though. If you have a real medical concern, or if something serious or immediate is wrong with your child, put this book down and go call your doctor. I'm not here to actually diagnose, treat, or cure your child of anything.

Basically, this book is for common sense. If your child wakes up with the sniffles, check out some basic remedies that could help ease them so s/he can sleep more peacefully. If your child is actually having trouble breathing, go call a doctor.

Or, if your child is a picky eater and you need some help devising kid-friendly real-food meals, check the food section of this book. If your child has a serious eating disorder and is very over or under-weight, get him/her to a doctor.

Make sense?

Just so we're all on the same page...figuratively and literally. J This book is intended to help parents in the day-to-day aspects of raising a healthy child. It's not meant to be able to address serious health concerns. And we've even included a section on "when to call the doctor," just in case you have any hesitations at all if what you're dealing with is really serious.

Enjoy, and I hope it helps you raise healthy children!

HOW TO USE THIS BOOK

This book is broken down into three sections: food, health, and environment.

In the food section, you'll find advice on what to feed your children, how to help older kids with the transition to a new way of eating, dealing with pickiness, meal and snack ideas, getting kids involved in food preparation, and a few kid-friendly real food recipes. It also addresses a few common questions, like about milk (good? Bad? What kind?) and grains. This section is intended to help you feed your children well with real, whole foods.

In the health section, you'll find many of the common concerns parents have about health: when to see a doctor, what about the vaccine debate, how to treat common acute illnesses at home, some natural ideas to support chronic illnesses (this does not replace consultation/management by a medical professional), an herbal guide, and alternative medicine options. If you need an overview of what "natural medicine" looks like and are seeking some safe home remedies for common, acute illnesses, you'll find them here.

In the final section, we have environment. This means clothing, bedding, bath products, keeping the home allergy-free, and similar subjects. Basically anything in the environment! There are a couple brief sections on TV/media and positive discipline, although child-rearing practices are not the focus of this book. They are included because a lot of parents have questions about them! See the 'resources' page if you have additional questions about these or any other subjects.

Check the table of contents for your concern, then flip to the appropriate section or page. And remember that the book can't diagnose, treat, or cure anything serious; it's for informational purposes only.

RESOURCES

Food

- *Real Food: What to Eat and Why* by Nina Planck
- *Nourishing Traditions* by Sally Fallon and Mary Enig
- *The Nourishing Traditions Book of Baby & Child Care* by Sally Fallon and Thomas Cowan
- *Healing Our Children* by Sally Fallon and Ramiel Nagel

Health

- *How to Raise a Healthy Child In Spite of Your Doctor* by Dr. Robert Mendelssohn
- *The Vaccine Book* by Dr. Robert Sears
- *Rosemary Gladstar's Herbal Remedies for Children's Health* by Rosemary Gladstar
- *Vaccine Free: 111 Stories of Unvaccinated Children* by Andreas Bachmair
- *Vaccines: Are They Really Safe and Effective* by Neil Z. Miller
- *What Your Doctor May Not Tell You About Children's Vaccinations* by Dr. Stephanie Cave and Deborah Mitchell
- *Herbal Healing for Children* by Demetria Clark
- *Gut and Psychology Syndrome* by Dr. Natasha Campbell-McBride
- *Naturally Healthy Babies and Children: A Commonsense Guide to Herbal Remedies, Nutrition, and Health* by Aviva Jill Romm and William Sears
- *Curing Tooth Decay* by Ramiel Nagel

Environment

- *Positive Discipline* by Jane Nelsen
- *Positive Discipline A – Z: 1001 Solutions to Everyday Parenting Problems*, by Jane Nelsen, Ed.D
- *How to Talk so Kids will Listen & Listen so Kids Will Talk* by Adele Faber and Elaine Mazlish

DISCLAIMER

This book is not written by a medical professional. It is not intended to diagnose, treat, or cure any disease or condition. It has not been reviewed or endorsed by the FDA or any other major medical body. It is a guide written by a mom, for moms. It's intended to be well-researched and helpful, but it's not medical advice and shouldn't be viewed as such.

If you have any specific concerns about your child's health or believe that your child's situation may be serious, please seek the advice of a qualified medical professional immediately. This book is meant for acute, self-limiting situations only and is not a substitute for medical advice. Please ask your doctor if you have any specific questions or concerns.

SECTION 1: FOOD

WHY NUTRITION IS SO IMPORTANT

A book on health wouldn't be complete without a thorough discussion on nutrition. These days, there is so little respect for the role that good nutrition plays. Most think that if children are eating some fruits and vegetables, low-fat proteins, and plenty of milk (with not too much sugar or fat) that they're doing just fine. Too many parents fall for labeling gimmicks at the store that are not intended to help families make healthy choices, but are really intended to sell products (see the section on Food Label Tricks later).

Most people acknowledge that eating healthy food can help kids to grow up big and strong. But after that, it gets muddled. What *is* good nutrition? What food is actually healthy? And can food do more than just meet our basic needs for energy, growth, and development?

The truth is, nutrition affects nearly everything we do. Our bodies rely on optimal nutrition in order to function. Children rely on nutrition even more heavily because they *are* growing and changing so rapidly (and this is most evident in the first couple years and the teen years). Vitamin deficiencies during development can affect so many body systems.

Vitamin deficiencies have been tied to:

- Asthma (deficiencies in A, C, and D)[1],[2]
- Allergies (deficiencies in D)[3],[4]
- Autism (deficiencies in D)[5],[6]
- ADHD (deficiencies in magnesium)[7]
- Learning disabilities (deficiencies in C, D)[8],[9]
- Hypothyroidism (deficiencies in A, B12)[10],[11]
- Obesity (deficiencies in calcium, D, dietary fat)[12],[13]
- Diabetes, type 1 and 2 (deficiencies in B12, D, K)[14],[15],[16],[17]

1   http://www.rodale.com/asthma-and-vitamins
2   http://www.sciencedaily.com/releases/2011/09/110922134540.htm
3   http://www.myhealthnewsdaily.com/992-vitamin-d-allergies-linked-in-kids-110224.html
4   http://www.medicalnewstoday.com/releases/213251.php
5   http://www.scientificamerican.com/article.cfm?id=vitamin-d-and-autism
6   http://www.sciencedirect.com/science/article/pii/S0891422212000431
7   http://www.ncbi.nlm.nih.gov/pubmed/16846100
8   http://autismjabberwocky.blogspot.com/2012/03/study-maternal-vitamin-d-deficiency.html
9   http://www.sciencedaily.com/releases/2009/09/090902112115.htm
10 http://www.ithyroid.com/vitamin_a.htm
11 http://www.ncbi.nlm.nih.gov/pubmed/18655403
12 http://www.ncbi.nlm.nih.gov/pubmed/19054627
13 http://people.csail.mit.edu/seneff/obesity_epidemic.html
14 http://www.jabfm.org/content/22/5/528.abstract
15 http://www.sciencedaily.com/releases/2012/07/120717162738.htm
16 http://ucsdnews.ucsd.edu/pressrelease/vitamin_d_deficiency_linked_to_type_1_diabetes
17 http://www.nutraingredients-usa.com/Research/Vitamin-K-may-slash-diabetes-risk-Study

- Anemia (deficiencies in iron, B12, D)[18],[19],[20]

It's obvious that vitamin deficiencies – especially B12 andD – are heavily related to many of the common ailments children are dealing with today!

Although levels can be raised from severely deficient to "acceptable," lowering risk a bit by using synthetic supplements, the ideal place to get nutrients is from food. Nourishing children can potentially prevent the above conditions, as well as helping them to develop strong bones, muscles, and overall body systems. It may even help to raise their IQ[21].

We cannot dismiss the critical importance that diet plays in nourishing our children. A nourishing diet is one which is free from as many processed foods as possible and which includes nutrient-dense, full fat options like bone broth, raw and full-fat dairy, fruits, vegetables, soaked whole grains, and other foods in their unprocessed state. Continue reading for more information about why these foods are so healthy!

The variety of processed "healthy" options available on store shelves are not, in fact, healthy, and should largely be avoided. In later sections we will look at super foods, ingredients to avoid, and tricky labeling techniques used to get parents to buy not-so-healthy processed options.

18   http://iron.sabm.org/overview/docs/laboratory_studies_in_the_diagnosis_of_iron_deficiency.pdf
19   http://www.ahealthstudy.com/diseases/vitamin-b12-deficiency-anemia
20   http://www.ncbi.nlm.nih.gov/pmc/articles/PMC2840674/
21   http://www.sciencedaily.com/releases/2012/08/120807095740.htm

10 SUPER FOODS FOR KIDS

Let's face it. Sometimes it's hard to figure out what the best foods are to serve to kids. And among them, foods kids will actually *eat*. As adults we can sometimes talk ourselves into eating something because it's "good for us" even if we don't care for it. With kids, that's a hard sell.

These are 10 super foods that most kids will really eat...and some suggestions for serving them in even more kid-friendly ways.

#1: Bone broth

Why: Bone broth keeps you healthy! It pulls impurities out of the gut and helps to heal and seal any openings in the gut. It may help prevent or ease the symptoms of a cold or flu. It also contains calcium, magnesium, zinc, and other important minerals.

How to serve: In favorite soup recipes, or cook veggies, potatoes or rice in it for reluctant eaters.

#2: Raw cheese

Why: Raw, grass-fed dairy products are a powerhouse of nutrition and a complete food. Usually a kid-favorite too! It contains calcium and vitamin D.

How to serve: Plain cubes, or lightly melted on crackers or veggies, or on pizza or in soups.

#3: Soaked, dehydrated nut butters

Why: Store-bought nut butters have anti-nutrients, but soaked and dehydrated versions are extremely healthy and kid-friendly. They pack protein, healthy fat, and a lot of other nutrients.

How to serve: On sandwiches, crackers, as a dip with veggies, mixed into healthy "fudge" and more.

#4: Plain yogurt

Why: Full-fat yogurt is full of protein, healthy fat, and probiotics. Kids need all of these!

How to serve: By itself, if your kid will eat it. If not, add some fresh berries and a drizzle of honey, or use it as the base for a fruit smoothie.

#5: Avocado

Why: Full of healthy fats and plenty of vitamins and minerals, as well as healthy monounsaturated fats! Also an excellent first food for babies.

How to serve: Plain chunks or slices on top of burgers or tacos; made into guacamole; for picky eaters, mix with honey and chocolate to make "pudding."

#6: Bananas

Why: Bananas are very sweet and easy to take along. They're filled with potassium that growing kids need, along with lots of nutrients!

How to serve: By themselves, on a nut butter and honey sandwich, turned into muffins or bread, in smoothies, or even dipped in chocolate.

#7: Pastured Meats

Why: Pastured meats are from animals allowed to truly free-range, and they contain high levels of CLA, B vitamins, iron, and other needed nutrients, plus lots of protein.

How to serve: Make homemade chicken nuggets, burgers, meatballs, or serve in whatever form your child likes.

#8: Eggs

Why: Eggs are a great source of B vitamins, choline, and other major nutrients. They're also rich in cholesterol (which is *good* for kids), especially if pastured.

How to serve: Scrambled, fried, hardboiled, or, for picky eaters, make coconut or almond flour baked goods that use lots of eggs. Custards and ice cream are other great ways.

#9: Soaked Whole Grains

Why: Whole grains are a good source of fiber, protein, B vitamins, and more. Soaking ensures that the phytic acid is gone or reduced (an anti-nutrient) and the nutrients are easily absorbed.

How to serve: As tortillas, waffles, pizza, English muffins, or any other preferred bread item.

#10: Raw honey and real maple syrup

Why: Although too much sugar is not good for anyone, these two are natural and contain enzymes to boost immunity and plenty of B vitamins and trace minerals. Small amounts are beneficial.

How to serve: In herbal tea, raw ice cream, on waffles, on crackers, etc.

Bonus super foods: oranges, lemons, blueberries, mushrooms, spinach, fermented veggies, beans, cooked tomatoes, broccoli.

Ideally, serve your child as many of these super foods as possible per day. Don't worry about the calories or number of servings; if they are eating healthy foods, allow them to eat until they are satisfied.

You may also be wondering why there are only a few fruits and veggies on this list. Many young children do not care for them, first of all. Also, they are harder to digest (especially raw) and children are unable to gain all the nutritional benefits from them. The fruits and veggies that are listed are easier to digest and are beneficial to children. This is up until age 5 or so.

If your child really likes fruits and veggies – I have a 3-year-old who loves salad – by all means, feed it to them! The list is meant to be super foods that are easily digestible and usually preferred by kids. There's nothing more frustrating than a list that's mostly beans, spinach, mushrooms (which are also super foods) that you know your kid won't eat! When you do serve fruits and veggies, pairing them with nut butters, real whipped cream, cooking them in stock or soups, etc. is a great idea. A little fat helps children to digest and absorb the nutrients more easily[22].

---

22   http://www.purdue.edu/newsroom/research/2012/120619FerruzziSalad.html

SHOULD YOU CHOOSE ORGANIC?

In late 2012, the AAP[23] came out with a statement on organic food. The gist was that although the pesticides used in conventional food production have been shown to be neurotoxic and carcinogenic (causes cancer), there's no "real proof" that these foods are healthier, so parents shouldn't make it a priority to buy them.

This is a pretty silly position for a number of reasons.

First, they are calling for double-blind, placebo-controlled studies to definitively "prove" that conventional foods are more dangerous to health. These studies are impossible. Pregnant women would have to be separated and fed an identical diet, and their children would have to be fed an identical diet also for several years – that means being offered the same foods in each group everyday, one group conventional and one organic – and they would also have to completely control for environmental factors like outside pollution, personal care products, medications, etc. There is no ethical or logical way to accomplish such a study.

Second, rather than calling for ridiculous studies, we should err on the side of caution and choose foods with fewer pesticides whenever possible. We should not give these chemicals the benefit of the doubt, especially since it has been shown in studies that children who eat conventional produce have the pesticides in their urine (suggesting that the produce remains contaminated).

Third, a lot of the industry studies[24] showing that the conventional foods and organic foods were equally nutritious weren't done fairly. They compared foods grown at a university in identical soil conditions, and tested their nutrient levels. But this soil was already depleted, so they came out the same. In a *true* organic environment, it isn't simply "a lack of pesticides," it's an integrative system that includes natural fertilizers, compost, and other natural elements to increase the nutrients in the soil. This test was not accurate for a real-world setting, in other words.

The basic idea is that yes, you should choose organic, if you possibly can.

Not everyone will have access to organic or be able to afford it, however. That is a consideration as well.

If possible, choose foods from the "dirty dozen[25]" list organic: apples, bell peppers, celery, grapes, blueberries, strawberries, potatoes, lettuce, green beans, spinach, nectarines, cucumbers.

Choose also foods that are fairly inexpensive organic: carrots, celery, lettuce, potatoes (this may vary depending on your area, but this is what I find cheaply in the mid-west).

Choose foods that are low on the pesticide residue list conventional (or those with a thick/inedible skin): avocado, lemon, lime, orange, mushrooms, onions, sweet corn (unless GMO), peas, broccoli, pineapple.

---

23   http://www.aap.org/en-us/about-the-aap/aap-press-room/Pages/American-Academy-of-Pediatrics-Weighs-In-For-the-First-Time-on-Organic-Foods-for-Children.aspx

24   http://www.tendergrassfedmeat.com/2012/09/04/when-organic-tests-no-better-check-the-soil-and-the-bias/

25   http://www.ewg.org/foodnews/list/

Don't be afraid to buy frozen if that's what's cheaper for you. We choose to buy a lot of frozen veggies especially during the winter months. Frozen veggies are great in soups, stews, casseroles, and so on.

Know the facts, then do the best you can.

There is also the issue of animal foods. While "organic" is certainly better here (it means the animals can't have been fed with grains containing GMOs, and they can't use growth hormones and antibiotic use is strictly regulated as a treatment, not a preventative), it's not indicative of high-quality.

The highest quality animal products are those which can be purchased directly from farms or local butchers. The animals should be raised on pasture as much as possible – ideally, sheep and cows should be 100% pastured, including at the end of their lives. There is a common practice of "finishing" cows on grains in feedlots for the last month or two of their lives to fatten them up. This should be avoided if possible.

These guidelines go not only for meat, but also for eggs, milk, butter, and any other animal products as well. Check www.eatwild.com for local sources near you, or visit a local farmer's market if there is one. Some major cities even have "winter markets" available now, and what is there is largely animal products (with some greenhouse produce or, if warm enough, seasonal fruits/veggies).

If you are unable to access local sources, then look for organic or at least hormone/antibiotic-free sources. The pesticides and any other toxins concentrate in the animal's fat (which is otherwise very healthy to consume) so every effort should be made to get better-quality animal products. If needed, consume less meat and make up the difference with beans, nuts, and grains – although these aren't as nourishing, especially for small children. Do what you can.

WHAT IF I HAVE A PICKY EATER?

Many parents dread meal times, because they know a battle will ensue. Some children are just a "little" picky – their food can't touch, it must be on the right color plate, etc. (but they'll eat most of it eventually). Other kids are *really* picky – there are only a few foods they will actually eat and anything else is entirely refused.

There are several possible reasons for a picky eater.

Food Intolerances

In my experience, seriously picky eaters are often picky due to food intolerances. Different foods make them not feel very well, so they refuse to eat them. Over time they suffer from gut damage[26] (like my oldest) and they self-limit to the foods that feed the "bad" bacteria in their systems: fruit, cheese, breads, and sugary foods[27]. If your child will literally only eat chicken nuggets, bread, pasta, cheese, and fruit – this may likely be what is going on. This is especially likely if they also suffer from eczema, diarrhea or constipation, sleep disturbances (frequent waking, night terrors), behavior issues (screaming, tantrums beyond what's developmentally appropriate; ADHD), etc.

If you suspect this may be a problem, the top culprits are dairy, gluten, soy, corn, seafood, although intolerances may be to just about anything. The best solution for children with serious issues is the GAPS diet[28], which we did with my oldest. She remains "picky" but not nearly what she was. (She does not like any sort of tomato product or sauce; but eats basically anything else.) It is not an easy or quick solution but it makes a world of difference long-term.

Processed Foods

Some parents have found that their children had developed a preference for certain sweet foods or certain types of processed foods and would not eat healthier foods as long as the processed options were available. Once they were switched to a diet of more "real food," they began to try new and interesting foods and flavors and actually enjoyed them.

In some cases children just don't like the processed version of a food but will enjoy the "real" version. i.e. children may dislike canned green beans, but serve them fresh green beans with bacon and they'll love it! If your children are picky but not seriously limiting their diets, try cooking healthy foods in new ways using whole, real ingredients. You may be surprised!

Lack of Variety

Some children appear picky because they have simply not had the opportunity to try many new foods at home. Some parents themselves are picky and do not serve foods they don't like. (My own mother doesn't eat any vegetables! My brother and I only learned to eat them because my father loved and often prepared them when we were older.) Coming across a new food for the first time at Grandma's house or a friend's house is more likely to lead to rejection than coming across a new food at home. Children also watch their parents – if the parents are avoiding it or do not seem to like

---

26   http://www.mcminnclinic.com/yeast-overgrowth/
27   http://www.mcminnclinic.com/yeast-overgrowth/
28   http://www.gapsdiet.com

it, children will be reluctant to even try. In contrast, if parents are enjoying the foods, children are more likely to want them! My children try the largest number of veggies when I am cutting them for a meal – they can't help but want to sample everything I chop!

Attempt to serve your kids more variety at home and to find new foods that you are willing to try yourself, if you are picky. Take the kids shopping with you and allow them to select new foods that they would like to try (fresh options, not prepared meals) and invite them into the kitchen to help you do so. When they are invested in the project, they are more likely to try the food.

What To Do in the Mean Time?

Some parents wonder what to do about their picky eater in the mean time. All of the above ideas take time.

It is possible to "hide" some healthy foods within other foods, although it's not my favorite tactic. Especially if there is a chance that the child could be avoiding a particular food because it makes him feel sick, hiding it to 'force' it is not a good idea. If you know that something doesn't bother your child, you can add it to other foods. Zucchini or stock can be added to spaghetti sauce, various shredded fruits or veggies in muffins, lots of fruits and veggies in smoothies, and so on.

It is also possible to find some new, yummy recipes to prepare foods, or to simply serve them in new ways. One of my kids won't eat mushrooms cooked in any form, but begs to eat them raw (and the same with many other veggies, actually). Perhaps *your* preferred recipe is not your child's. Often picky children prefer their foods "plain," so a plate of raw fruits and veggies or meat with no sauce may go over better than a gourmet dish.

Take stock of what your child actually eats. Is it really that bad, even if limited? If your child is willing to eat foods from every category, even if there isn't a lot of variety, it may not be worth the battle. Keep offering new options, but don't be afraid to allow the child to eat the favorites (assuming they are healthy). Strive for the super foods in one of the previous sections whenever possible.

In general, if you feed your children real food, make sure they get probiotics in some form, and address any gut health/allergy issues (if any), pickiness will fade in time. Don't make eating a battle in the mean time. Offer what there is and relax!

EXPLAINING DIETARY CHANGES TO OLDER KIDS

It's pretty easy to feed a kid real food if you start them out on it from day 1. But what about if you've just begun your journey and your kids are 2, 5, 10, even teens? Changing to a diet that is very different from what they're used to and forbidding foods they love may result in mutiny!

The small ones – the under 5 crowd – are easier, because they have had less time eating one way. They are also not yet in school and are less aware of any social pressure to eat certain foods. The older ones are more aware of social pressure and the "options" out there, so they're a little harder. There are still several ways to explain dietary changes to kids.

Be Honest

If you're changing things up in the middle, then you owe your kids an explanation. "Mom and Dad didn't know that this food wasn't the healthiest choice, but we have recently learned some new things. We would like to change what we eat so that we can all feel better and hopefully get sick less often. It's going to be hard for us, too, to try some new foods and have our favorites less often." Rather than taking a hard stance or giving a trite "It's good for you" answer, really be honest about your own feelings about just learning this information and how it will be hard to give up certain foods. If your kids see the changes as something the whole family is working through together, they'll be more likely to cooperate than if they feel it's something being shoved upon them.

Talk About Being Healthy

Regardless of your kids' age, talk about how important it is to be healthy. "We want to eat good foods so we can grow up big and strong. These foods are healthy and will help us do that." If your children are older, read some of the product labels at the grocery store and ask them if it sounds like food (many will not). Have them read labels for themselves. Write down some of the unusual-sounding ingredients and look them up online together. Some older children may really like researching the different nutrients the foods contain and how they benefit their bodies. The more your children feel empowered and a part of this decision, and the more knowledge they have, the more likely they are to get on board.

Make Homemade Treats

One thing that we *all* miss is having our old favorites. Rather than saying "No more cookies!" find recipes to make healthier cookies at home. Get recipes for cheese sauce, pizza, whatever else your kids like (my book *Real Food Basics* is great for these type of recipes). If your kids know that they can still have their favorites, simply made at home, they'll be much less likely to rebel. They can even get involved in helping make it! My own kids now say "Can we make a healthy one at home?" when they see something in a store or restaurant they'd like to have. This is a good thing.

Find New Favorites

As you're trying new foods and new recipes, help the kids get excited about all the amazing new flavors. Real food does taste better! Emphasize how much better it helps you all feel, too. Help the kids to enjoy the experience of eating these foods and finding new favorite options.

Relax, Sometimes

Many families choose to live by the 80/20 or 90/10 rule. That is, the majority of what they eat is going to be healthy, but sometimes they'll let it slide. If you let your children know that you won't be buying special treats anymore, but that if Grandma offers them something or they go to a friend's birthday party they can eat what's there, then they'll be more likely to accept the changes. Many older kids are worried about social situations and knowing that they can eat what their friends are eating on special occasions helps them.

Give Them a Choice

Take your kids shopping with you or ask them to help make a meal plan or list with you. Help them get excited about all the new foods they get to eat, rather than focusing on the ones they can't. Older children (pre-teens and teens) especially need to have a choice. These older kids will be in plenty of situations where they will be able to choose what to eat without you, and they need to feel ownership of the changes. Explore new recipes and food purchases together so that they can find items they really want. Small children can be encouraged to pick one or two interesting-looking (healthy) foods at the grocery store, like a new vegetable – then you can take it home and prepare it together.

The more you talk about the changes openly and give kids a chance to understand and participate in the changes, the better things will go. Kids are smart, and they like to feel included rather than "ordered." And if your goal is for your children to stick to the changes even once they're not with you, they will need to embrace them.

KEEPING KIDS FROM OBESITY

One major concern that parents have these days is keeping kids from obesity. And with good reason! These days, between 16 and 33% of kids and teens are overweight or obese[29]. This is roughly a 60% increase since 1990[30], which shows that the problem is getting sharply worse. Obese children and teens have about an 80% chance of becoming obese adults, so this is a problem that needs curbed, and quickly!

The way this has been treated is by pushing kids to eat "healthier" foods (according to the USDA Dietary Guidelines) and get more exercise. Studies show that kids have been eating more junk foods and snack foods and exercising less and less since the late 70s[31]. Despite these efforts, which in recent years have turned to school lunch reforms[32] (with a focus on fresh fruits and vegetables and low-fat milk and meats), national exercise programs, and a general focus on calorie and portion reduction[33], kids have continued to get heavier. Over two-thirds of adults are now overweight or obese[34]...so this is serious!

Unfortunately, mainstream medicine has little to offer in the way of help. The first USDA Dietary Guidelines came out in 1977[35]. At that time, only about 13% of people were obese. By 1997 it was 19%, and now it is about 36%[36] (a staggering increase in the last 15 years). The mainstream doctors blame this increase on junk food manufacturers, portion sizes, and peoples' unwillingness to follow USDA guidelines.

The evidence, however, shows that the guidelines (and available "food" options) just don't work. Despite continued harping on the food "pyramid" and now the "food plate[37]" people are getting heavier and sicker.

Concerned parents are restricting their kids' calorie and fat intakes and trying to feed them "healthy" packaged meal options. This is not going to help!

Kids need full-fat dairy, meat with fat on it, and no calorie restrictions. Studies show those who consume full-fat dairy weigh less[38], and children especially need fat for their developing brains. The brain is largely composed of fat[39], so depriving a child is going to affect brain development. Studies show that restricting a child's saturated fat intake doesn't lead to a reduction in the risk of obesity, but it does increase the risk of serious fat-soluble vitamin deficiencies, a real problem in developing children[40].

Instead of treating kids the same way as we have treated adults (which has resulted in heavier, sicker adults and is doing the same for children), we need to go back to a diet

29   http://www.aacap.org/cs/root/facts_for_families/obesity_in_children_and_teens
30   http://www.hsph.harvard.edu/obesity-prevention-source/obesity-trends/global-obesity-trends-in-children/index.html
31   http://aspe.hhs.gov/health/reports/child_obesity/
32   http://www.theatlanticwire.com/politics/2010/12/president-obama-signs-child-nutrition-act/21903/
33   http://www.ces.ncsu.edu/depts/fcs/pdfs/AO%20.pdf
34   http://www.cdc.gov/nchs/data/databriefs/db01.pdf
35   http://www.nal.usda.gov/fnic/pubs/bibs/gen/DGA.pdf
36   http://en.wikipedia.org/wiki/Obesity_in_the_United_States
37   http://www.choosemyplate.gov/
38   http://phys.org/news176467332.html
39   http://www.fi.edu/learn/brain/fats.html#fatsbuild
40   http://depts.washington.edu/mchprog/docs/posters/2010/GardnerCapstone.pdf

of whole foods. Fruits and vegetables, plain meats, whole grains (properly prepared), full-fat dairy (preferably raw) and so on. We need to avoid sugar, sugar substitutes, food additives, dyes, pesticides, and other industrial "foods." It is so important to feed kids real food. A child who eats real food and is encouraged to exercise regularly (believe me – they'll need to – real food kids have boundless energy!) will not become overweight.

It can even be detrimental psychologically to try to lay the burden of obesity and the 'necessity' of counting calories on a child. Children who are restricted in their eating and taught that healthy eating means restriction will grow up with an unhealthy attitude towards food, as well as potential body image issues. The focus should always be on health. A child who is allowed to self-regulate healthy food intake from birth will always be able to do so appropriately. Children generally go through phases, also, where they eat quite a lot (around growth spurts, both physical and mental) and other phases where they don't seem to need as much.

Should a real food kid become under or overweight, an underlying cause should be discussed with a doctor who is familiar with real food and who can check for metabolic issues or food intolerances that could be causing the problem. The same is true if a child seems truly unable to regulate his/her food intake for some reason – constantly eating, sneaking food, always wanting (and finding) sugary foods, etc. If your child's weight or food behavior is not normal, seek medical advice.

THE MILK QUESTION

How much milk should a child drink per day? What kind?

Most parents are very concerned with how much milk their children drink. Mainstream sources[41] say that children should drink about 2 cups of milk per day and have 3 total servings of dairy (which includes yogurt, cheese, etc.). They warn against getting both too little and too much. The general advice is that children from age 1 – 2 need to consume whole milk, and children after age 2 should consume 1% or skim milk to avoid too much fat. (We busted the myth in the previous section that low-fat dairy is protective against obesity and in fact the opposite is true.)

Children do not, in fact, need to "drink milk." The idea that a cup of milk with meals is best practice is simply untrue. That's not to say that children who enjoy milk should not be allowed to drink it, of course. Ideally a child will be breastfed for 2 – 3 years and this will supply most of his/her needs for milk. After that, milk can be treated as something to have sometimes; a part of a healthy diet, but by no means a panacea, an answer to picky eating.

---

41   http://www.parenting.com/article/got-milk

WHAT TYPE OF MILK?

Health-conscious parents want to know what kind of milk children should drink. The above recommendations are, of course, for typical cow's milk. However, some parents believe that cow's milk may be associated with asthma, allergies, and other conditions. Some children are also allergic to cow's milk or are lactose-intolerant. These parents often turn to alternatives like soy, almond, or coconut milk instead of cow's milk. Some also prefer goat's milk (which does have a closer nutrient profile to human milk, although it lacks B12).

Soy milk is problematic, especially if consumed in large quantities (and even more so if lots of other soy-based foods are consumed regularly). Soy has been shown to have a high phytoestrogen content, which has uncertain effects[42], but may be related to cancer in pre-pubescent children and may affect cell division and migration[43]. Because of these potential effects and general uncertainty, soy is best skipped.

Almond milk is another common choice. However, it has three major problems. If produced commercially, it usually contains carrageenan, guar gum, or other food additives[44], which are better avoided. It is fairly low in beneficial fats[45], especially compared to whole cow's milk. Finally, it contains high levels of phytic acid, which can block nutrient absorption[46]. Nuts, for a select few, may also cause severe allergies. Although homemade almond milk from properly soaked almonds (soaking in a salt water solution overnight, then discarding the soaking water can decrease phytic acid) is not a bad idea on occasion, it should not be a staple of the diet.

Coconut milk is the ideal choice for those who need a dairy substitute. Coconut milk contains plenty of beneficial saturated fats[47], and also the medium-chain fatty acid lauric acid[48], which has a protective immune function[49]. Commercial coconut milk still contains undesirable additives[50], so the best solution is to make it at home[51]. There is one company that makes it without additives although it is more expensive[52].

However, the question of cow's milk hasn't been settled yet. Why not cow's milk? Research shows that there is no evidence currently that cow's milk actually increases the likelihood of asthma[53] (although it may worsen symptoms in a child who is dairy-allergic).

There are still reasons to be cautious about cow's milk, though, especially if store-bought. There is evidence to show that modern milking practices drive hormone levels to extreme heights, which may be linked to certain types of cancer[54] (and this does not include synthetic hormones introduced). There are even greater problems suspected

42   http://www.ncbi.nlm.nih.gov/pmc/articles/PMC1240881/pdf/ehp0110-a00294.pdf
43   http://www.ncbi.nlm.nih.gov/pmc/articles/PMC1257582/
44   http://www.bluediamond.com/index.cfm?navid=52
45   http://www.bluediamond.com/index.cfm?navid=52
46   http://chriskresser.com/another-reason-you-shouldnt-go-nuts-on-nuts
47   http://caloriecount.about.com/calories-coconut-milk-i12117
48   http://www.tiana-coconut.com/lauric_acid.html
49   http://www.jimmunol.org/content/174/9/5390.full
50   http://sodeliciousdairyfree.com/products/coconut-milk-beverages/original
51   http://wholenewmom.com/recipes/make-your-own-coconut-milk/
52   http://www.wildernessfamilynaturals.com/category/coconut-products-coconut-milk.php
53   http://www.wildernessfamilynaturals.com/category/coconut-products-coconut-milk.php
54   http://www.news.harvard.edu/gazette/2006/12.07/11-dairy.html

with the use of rbST and rBGH (synthetic hormones), although there are few studies proving anything[55]. These drugs have been shown to increase the need for antibiotics in cows who receive them. Antibiotics have been used increasingly over the last couple decades (rbST and rBGH were first approved in 1993) and are used in over 90% of all large farm operations[56]. This is theorized to cause antibiotic resistance in humans[57] (meaning that there are antibiotic residues in the milk we are consuming).

Large-scale farms are not the place to be buying milk! This milk is also pasteurized because it will make people sick otherwise – the use of hormones especially increases the risk of mastitis in cows and the possibility of pus in the milk[58]. Pasteurization may denature both casein and whey proteins in the milk and the effect this has is unknown[59] (although there is quite a bit of anecdotal evidence that people who are intolerant to pasteurized milk can consume unpasteurized milk without incident). Pasteurization also reduces vitamin C and several of the B vitamins, and may prevent the absorption of B-9, folate[60], which is needed to prevent neural tube defects in babies. Raw milk may be associated with a reduction in allergies[61].

A fairly recent study showed that raw milk drinkers have less allergies and asthma than pasteurized milk drinkers[62]. Raw milk has been associated in limited cases with infections like campylobacter and salmonella, but there is very little data showing how many illnesses are confirmed to be from a raw milk source. With an estimated 9 million regular drinkers and a tiny handful of suspected cases of illness each year, raw milk is not an overall dangerous food[63].

Raw milk is rich in enzymes, vitamins, minerals, and has been purported to help with a number of different health conditions. There are very few studies confirming or denying these but these anecdotal evidence is quite strong.

If you are unable to access raw milk, it is a toss-up whether organic milk or coconut milk will be better. Ideally, milk should not be ultra-pasteurized (which most organic milk is). It will depend on what is available to you and how your family reacts. Organic milk is "good" in that it doesn't contain antibiotics and hormones, but it's also not grass-fed and it is usually ultra-pasteurized. Try out both regular pasteurized organic milk and additive-free coconut milk to see what your family prefers and on what they feel the best.

In our personal experience, our older children were dairy intolerant to pasteurized milk, but have no issues with raw. We know many others personally who thrive on raw dairy who cannot tolerate pasteurized dairy. We even know a few who are so lactose intolerant that a small piece of milk chocolate would cause them severe distress; yet they can drink raw milk by the glass with no issue. This is anecdotal only but with a lack of scientific evidence available it is important.

55	http://www.gracelinks.org/797/rbgh
56	http://www.docstoc.com/docs/21076670/Antibiotic-Use-in-US-Livestock-Production-Summary-Antibiotics
57	http://www.cbsnews.com/stories/2007/03/11/eveningnews/main2556945.shtml
58	http://www.ejnet.org/bgh/nogood.html
59	http://ohioline.osu.edu/fse-fact/pdf/0003.pdf
60	http://www.ncbi.nlm.nih.gov/pubmed/7097350
61	http://www.ncbi.nlm.nih.gov/pubmed/22054181
62	http://www.reuters.com/article/2011/09/13/us-kids-raw-milk-idUSTRE78C75O20110913
63	http://www.foodrenegade.com/government-data-proves-raw-milk-safe/

The bottom line: while children do not *need* to drink large quantities of milk (and in fact doing so may lead to anemia[64] as calcium blocks iron absorption[65]), the best choices for dairy are raw milk or coconut milk.

If parents are simply looking for calcium for their children, it can be obtained from a number of different food sources[66], like: collard greens, salmon, almonds, oranges, bone broth[67], and more. It is possible to obtain all the necessary nutrients from non-dairy foods or from other forms of dairy (cheese, yogurt, kefir) instead of drinking plain milk.

64   http://www.nlm.nih.gov/medlineplus/ency/article/007134.htm
65   http://www.ncbi.nlm.nih.gov/pubmed/1600930
66   http://www.hsph.harvard.edu/nutritionsource/what-should-you-eat/calcium-sources/index.html
67   http://www.jadeinstitute.com/jade/bone-broth-health-building.php

GRAINS AND SUGAR: GOOD OR BAD?

As I began writing this book, I realized that the issue of grains was something I needed to address. A lot of "healthy eaters" have come to believe that all grains are bad, or certainly that all gluten is bad. Many, without evidence of intolerance, are striving to eat gluten or grain-free most of the time for "improved health." Is this really necessary, or beneficial, especially for children?

It's true that gluten intolerance has been increasing sharply over the last 50 to 60 years, and is thought to affect nearly 1% of the population now[68]. It is not, however, a well-researched area. Many doctors still believe that only those with celiac disease should truly avoid gluten; while others know that intolerance without celiac is possible. There *are* people out there who need to avoid gluten for one reason or another.

Some point to modern wheat breeding as a major reason for the rise in gluten intolerance[69]. A few go as far as to call modern wheat "poison" and suggest that people should never eat it. This is probably an overreaction for most.

A bigger concern than gluten, for many people, is phytic acid, which all grains, nuts, legumes, and seeds contain. Phytic acid binds with important nutrients and can prevent absorption and cause deficiency, especially in iron, zinc, calcium, and magnesium[70]. However, reducing phytic acid has been shown to negate this action and allow grains to provide the appropriate nutrients. Grains low in phytic acid have been associated with rebounding mineral levels[71].

Reducing the phytic acid, however, is fairly easy: soaking the grains before preparing them reduces the phytic acid levels fairly rapidly, with the exception of oats and corn[72]. Learning to properly soak can allow your family to consume whole grains without incident. The soaking process also breaks down some of the gluten, meaning that some of those with minor gluten intolerance can also consume the soaked breads that result.

The bottom line is that grains are not bad, but we should not rely too heavily on them (20 – 30% of the diet is good; 60% is too much) and they should be whole, unrefined grains that have been properly soaked.

As for sugar, we all know that too much is bad for us. Too much can affect brain function and impair learning ability[73]. It may increase the risk of heart disease[74]. High fructose corn syrup is even worse than regular white sugar; it leads to increased weight gain and all the risks associated with weight gain[75]. Most sugar in the U.S. comes from sugar beets, and is genetically modified[76]. There have been no studies proving that genetic modification of crops is safe in the long term. There is some evidence coming out now that GMO crops are, in fact, potentially dangerous to human health[77].

68   http://online.wsj.com/article/SB10001424052748704893604576200393522456636.html
69   http://www.ncbi.nlm.nih.gov/pubmed/20664999
70   http://jn.nutrition.org/content/133/9/2973S.long
71   http://jn.nutrition.org/content/133/9/2973S.long
72   http://www.rebuild-from-depression.com/soaking-grains
73   http://www.sciencedaily.com/releases/2012/05/120515150938.htm
74   http://www.time.com/time/health/article/0,8599,1983542,00.html
75   http://www.princeton.edu/main/news/archive/S26/91/22K07/
76   http://www.rodaleinstitute.org/20110206_USDA-approves-genetically-engineered-sugar-beets
77   http://responsibletechnology.org/fraud/rigged-studies/Genetically-Modified-Corn-Study-Reveals-Health-Damage-and-Cover-up-June-2005

Even if this weren't true, sugar contains no nutrients or nutritional value of its own, but does require the body to use up sodium, magnesium, potassium, and calcium in order to metabolize it – which is why some call it an anti-nutrient[78]. Regular consumption of any sort of refined sugar is a poor choice in the diet.

Real maple syrup is high in manganese, B vitamins, and also contains lower amounts of other trace minerals[79]. While consuming it in large quantities is not advisable, a small amount used to sweeten treats is fine.

Raw honey, too, is a good option. It contains nutrients like magnesium, potassium, sodium, calcium, copper, iron, manganese, sulfur, zinc, phosphate, and B vitamins[80]. It has shown to have some beneficial effect on gut flora, specifically the bifidobacterium strain[81] (which is good). Honey has been shown to be beneficial in wound care due to its natural antibacterial properties[82],[83]. It must be consumed raw, on a spoon or in warm tea, and not baked with, to retain these properties.

There is also sucanat, which stands for "sugar cane natural." It is simply dried, granulated sugar cane that has not been refined. It contains a number of trace minerals, like calcium, magnesium, zinc, iron, phosphorus, potassium, and copper[84]. It, too, is acceptable in small amounts.

Ideally sugar in general is limited to only a teaspoon or two per day, but a treat now and then made with the above whole sweeteners isn't going to ruin a child. Being able to have a treat, especially when faced with a myriad of unhealthy options may even be beneficial socially because the child will not feel deprived. Don't be afraid to make the occasional homemade treat.

In general, grains and sugar require moderation and choosing an unprocessed option, but can be included in a healthy diet.

---

78   http://www.macrobiotics.co.uk/sugar.htm
79   http://www.purecanadamaple.com/benefits-of-maple-syrup/maple-syrup-nutrition/
80   http://www.purecanadamaple.com/benefits-of-maple-syrup/maple-syrup-nutrition/
81   http://www.ebeehoney.com/assets/images/PDFs/honeybifido.pdf
82   http://www.ncbi.nlm.nih.gov/pubmed/19222654
83   http://www.jcasonline.com/article.asp?issn=0974-2077;year=2011;volume=4;issue=3;spage=183;e
        page=187;aulast=Gupta
84   http://www.purcellmountainfarms.com/Organic%20Sucanat.htm

SPECIAL DIETS

Some children, for one reason or another, need to be on a special diet. There are many special diets out there, many driven by allergies. Children may be on gluten-free diet, or a dairy-free diet, or they may have multiple allergies. This doesn't make eating away from home – or even *at* home – very easy.

First, check out the sections on Food Label Tricks and Ingredients to Avoid at the Store so that at least eating at home isn't so difficult. For those with severe issues, restaurants may need to be avoided entirely, or a 'safe list' for your family may need to be developed. Although not especially healthy, we've found that Buffalo Wild Wings has a fairly extensive allergen menu. Not all restaurants are nearly as transparent. Organic/local restaurants may be a good bet in some cases as well – we are lucky to have some selections near us. There is more information on allergies in later sections.

Although there are many types of special diets, there are two in particular that I want to mention, as many parents may not be familiar with them.

Feingold Diet

This diet is intended to help children who are suffering from ADHD and other attention issues. The diet centers around removing artificial flavors and colors, artificial sweeteners, preservatives like BHT, plus salicylates[85]. (Salicylates are added back in slowly later on the diet, as they are found in unprocessed foods, but may cause a reaction in some children.) The idea is that the negative reactions to these chemicals cause a child to behave in a hyperactive manner.

The diet is not too difficult to follow if unprocessed foods are eaten. For those who are new to the idea of unprocessed or homemade foods, it may be overwhelming at first. Artificial colors, flavors, and preservatives are found in many foods. See the link to read more about the diet.

GAPS Diet

This diet is intended to heal gut damage in children, which may result in autism, ADHD, severe food allergies, or other outward symptoms. Children who have severe physical and behavioral problems may begin this diet in order to address the underlying causes, which is a so-called "leaky gut." This means that the good gut flora that should be present isn't, and that there are "holes" in the gut wall where undigested proteins are leaking through and into the bloodstream, sensitizing the child. There is also an overgrowth of pathogenic bacteria and likely, candida.

The GAPS diet[86] addresses this and helps to actually heal the gut. First, it removes all sugars (except honey), limits fruit, and removes all grains and complex starches. That means no seeds, no wheat, oats, spelt, potatoes, and so on. The diet focuses on non-starchy vegetables, meats, bone broth, fats, and probiotics. Broth is used to provide nutrients and to help pull the "junk" out of the body. Fats nourish the body and are soothing to the gut. Probiotics (good bacteria) re-seed the gut with friendly bacteria. Most of the early diet is soups.

Some people have to use digestive enzymes, enemas (water), and other additives early

---

85   http://www.feingold.org/overview.php
86   http://www.gapsdiet.com

on. Many choose to use a probiotic supplement in addition to probiotic foods, which should be included with every meal.

The diet is not easy, especially for someone just starting out. It can cause severe detox, including lethargy, vomiting, lack of appetite, headaches, and more. This is a sign of needing to back off a bit temporarily. Drinking ginger tea and taking baths with Epsom salts daily or even between every meal can help quite a lot to ease the detox reaction.

Most people are on the diet from six months to three years. It is intended as a temporary, healing diet – not a long-term lifestyle. At the end of the diet, the person slowly transitions back to eating fruits, properly soaked or sprouted grains, and so on. After the healing, these foods usually don't cause a reaction any longer.

There are many stories of children actually healing from autism, enough to lose their official diagnosis, by using this diet. It is worth it for those whose lives are severely affected by physical and behavioral symptoms.

While special diets are never easy, especially while out and about, they are worth it to those who need the help.

INGREDIENTS TO AVOID AT THE STORE

When purchasing food for your family, the goal is obviously to get the best quality food available without spending an arm and a leg. Ideally, families should seek local farms to purchase from, especially for animal products (meat, eggs, milk). Still, no matter what, families typically need to buy some items from regular grocery stores. And sometimes those purchases will be convenience items, because of time or money constraints.

This leaves a small problem: which ingredients are okay, and which are not? Ingredient lists should be as short as possible and should be largely or entirely recognizable as actual food. This eliminates about 99% of all products. Which ingredients *really* need to be avoided...and why?

The ones that I would consider "very bad" and which should always be avoided are marked with *.

Important: *Most* of these can be found in products at health food stores! Only a very small fraction have been banned (HFCS, artificial colors and flavors, sometimes artificial sweeteners). All other additives are easily and frequently found in health food store products. Read the labels *everywhere* you go and do not assume.

Artificial flavors* – These are laboratory-made chemical compositions used to flavor food. They are often petroleum-derived. Some have been implicated in the development of chronic illnesses[87]. They may also negatively impact a child's behavior[88] [89].

Aspartame* – This is an artificial sweetener that is found in many baked goods and other processed products. It is most famously in diet soda. It has been linked to obesity, cancer, and various other serious health concerns[90].

Autolyzed yeast extract* – It is made from growing yeast and then having it "digest" itself, then is washed with water to form an extract. It contains quite a bit of MSG, and may contain gluten, causing sensitivity issues in a number of individuals[91].

BHA* – This is used as a preservative in some types of oils and solid fats, and it is carcinogenic[92] (causes cancer).

BHT* – This is also used as a preservative, and some studies show an association with fatty livers and unusual cellular activity[93].

Canola oil – This is an oil derived from the rapeseed (which generally is toxic to humans). It is high in polyunsaturated fatty acids and omega-6s. It is also known to deplete vitamin E, a critical fat-soluble vitamin[94].

Caramel color* – This is a form of coloring used in sodas and other food products, and research has shown it to be carcinogenic[95].

---

87   http://www.sciencedaily.com/releases/2012/08/120801132606.htm
88   http://www.chem-tox.com/pregnancy/artificial.htm
89   http://www.feingold.org/Research/adhd.html
90   http://www.feingold.org/Research/adhd.html
91   http://www.quora.com/Will-autolyzed-yeast-extract-conflict-with-Celiac-disease
92   http://ntp.niehs.nih.gov/ntp/roc/twelfth/profiles/ButylatedHydroxyanisole.pdf
93   http://www.feingold.org/Research/bht.html
94   http://customers.hbci.com/~wenonah/new/canola.htm
95   http://www.huffingtonpost.com/michael-f-jacobson/caramel-coloring-in-soda-_b_823639.html

Carrageenan – This is a "gummy" substance used to improve the viscosity of different products. It is similar to plastic and has been linked to cancer[96].

Corn oil(– Corn oil is extremely high in omega-6s and is usually derived from GMO corn. It has been linked to certain forms of cancer[97].

Corn syrup* – This is a liquid sweetener made from corn, and it's largely GMO.

FD&C colors* – These dyes are derived from coal tar and petroleum, and have been linked to hyperactivity, reproductive issues (infertility), DNA changes, cancer, and many other scary issues[98].

Guar gum – This is a food additive that is a form of fiber. There are mixed results on this, but it may change the way nutrients are absorbed and in large doses could block the digestive tract[99].

High fructose corn syrup* – This is largely made from GMO corn, and is treated with enzymes to specifically make it higher in fructose than glucose. It has been shown to cause weight gain[100] and is associated with cancer[101].

Hydrogenated oils* – These are man-made oils (hydrogen is added to make the fat more solid, which increases its shelf life) and have been linked to high cholesterol and heart disease[102].

Modified corn starch* – This is an enzyme-modified starch used to thicken foods. There is no specific evidence that it is harmful, but it is usually GMO and is stripped of all actual nutrients.

Modified food starch* – This may be cornstarch, or it may be derived from wheat, potatoes, or another starchy food. It is used similarly to modified corn starch, to thicken foods, and is nutritionally devoid.

MSG* – This is a food additive (different from the naturally-occurring free glutamic acid, an amino acid in many foods) that has been linked to migraines, kidney and liver damage, learning disabilities, and a lot more[103].

Natural flavors – These are flavors that are originally derived from a natural substance, but which may have been chemically altered and simplified and tested to be "safe." They are not actually natural.

Potassium Sorbate – This is a preservative used to inhibit mold growth in food, and has been linked to DNA changes[104].

Sodium Benzoate* – This is another preservative, and when mixed with vitamin C, forms benzene, a toxic substance[105]. It has also been associated with infertility[106].

96   http://blog.healthkismet.com/carrageenan-cancer-health-inflammation
97   http://www.ncbi.nlm.nih.gov/pubmed/12616305
98   http://www.feingold.org/dye-studies.html
99   http://www.ranteccorp.com/MSDS%20PDFs/Guar%20Gum%20MSDS.pdf
100   http://www.ranteccorp.com/MSDS%20PDFs/Guar%20Gum%20MSDS.pdf
101   http://www.reuters.com/article/2010/08/02/cancer-fructose-idAFN0210830520100802
102   http://www.hsph.harvard.edu/nutritionsource/nutrition-news/transfats/
103   http://www.feingold.org/Research/msg.html
104   http://theorganicsinstitute.com/tag/potassium-sorbate/
105   http://theorganicsinstitute.com/tag/potassium-sorbate/
106   http://www.inchem.org/documents/cicads/cicads/cicad26.htm#SubSectionNumber:8.5.2

Soybean oil – Soy is high in phytoestrogens, is usually GMO, and the oil is high in omega-6s and polyunsaturated fatty acids[107]. This is best skipped.

Soy lecithin – Chemical solvents are used to "de-gum" soybean oil; the resulting "gummy" substance is soy lecithin. While lecithin is an essential nutrient, this GMO, chemically-processed version is not healthy[108].

Textured vegetable protein – This is soy-derived, usually GMO, and heavily processed. It has the issues associated with soy (causing early puberty and affecting fertility), and it also contains gluten[109].

Splenda (sucralose)* – This is an artificial sweetener that is said to be "made from sugar," but it contains chlorine, and has been associated with cancer and a number of other serious side effects[110].

Whey protein – Whey protein is extracted from dairy. It is processed at high heat and dried. It may contain MSG due to the processing, and it could contain hormones from the dairy source. Plus, access protein consumption places a strain on the liver and kidneys[111].

Xanthan gum – This is a fermentation of a sugar solution, extracted with isopropyl alcohol. There is some evidence that inhalation damages lungs, and it may increase the risk of aspiration in certain people when used to thicken foods[112].

Now that you are aware of common ingredients, try to avoid them when possible! Some are clearly worse than others. When possible, don't buy processed foods. When you need something easy or a treat, look for "better" options and avoid those with the worst ingredients.

---

107   http://www.westonaprice.org/soy-alert/studies-showing-adverse-effects-of-soy
108   http://www.westonaprice.org/soy-alert/studies-showing-adverse-effects-of-soy
109   http://www.livestrong.com/article/542141-what-are-the-dangers-of-texturized-vegetable-protein-tvp/
110   http://www.livestrong.com/article/542141-what-are-the-dangers-of-texturized-vegetable-protein-tvp/
111   http://www.musclebuildingdaily.com/supplements/whey-protein-dangers.php
112   http://en.wikipedia.org/wiki/Xanthan_gum

FOOD LABEL TRICKS

If you walk into any grocery store, you'll see lots of labels screaming at you "No artificial colors or flavors!" "100% juice!" "A Good Source Of ____!"

The thing is...these labels are not a good way to make decisions about healthy foods. They are labeling tricks to get you to buy products. It's called marketing, and it can't be trusted to guide you towards the truly healthy products.

Ideally, the majority of the products you purchase do not come with labels, or have only single-ingredient labels (i.e. fresh fruits, veggies, meats, etc.). These products usually do not carry the bright, screaming labels.

However, sometimes it's nice to just buy some snacks or something to make life easier. And that's where these labeling tricks come into play (for the most part). In a few cases, there are even misleading labels on natural products. Let's take a look.

"Grass Fed Meat!" – In general, certain meats, like chicken should not be "grass fed." Chickens ought to be eating bugs and worms as well. As far as beef, grass-fed is best, but what matters is that they are grass-*finished*. That is, that they have been fed only grass throughout their lives. Technically companies can claim "grass-fed" even if that is only 30% of the animal's diet. There's a big difference in nutrition levels depending on exactly what the animal was fed. Don't necessarily believe this claim.

"Vegetarian-Fed" – This usually applies to eggs, and it means that chickens weren't given any animal by-products. That's good, but it usually also means they weren't given access to outdoors where they ate bugs and worms, either. This label doesn't guarantee good eggs.

"Cage-Free" – This applies to eggs and sometimes chickens. This just means they weren't raised in cages, but it doesn't mean that they had any access to the outdoors. Most cage-free chickens are kept in extremely crowded chicken houses that are really no better.

"A Good Source Of _____" – To be given this label, a product needs only carry 10% of the RDA per serving. This isn't a very high amount of any single vitamin or mineral and honestly does not make it "a good source of" anything. Plus, the nutrients might be synthetic (and therefore poorly absorbed), and the product could still contain plenty of not-so-great ingredients.

"Fortified with Vitamins and Minerals!" – This claim may take various different forms (for example, noting which vitamins and minerals it's fortified with), but what it means is "this product contains synthetic nutrients." This is not going to be well absorbed and does not make the product healthy. As with the previous claim, it may also contain a lot of undesirable ingredients (think of a popular chocolate milk mix).

"Low fat" – Most people still believe that low-fat is healthy, but it isn't. This claim really doesn't mean anything.

"No artificial colors or flavors" – It may still contain 'natural flavors' or other undesirable ingredients, so don't be fooled. It can often contain colors which may or may not be natural as well, like annatto.

"No high fructose corn syrup" – It may still contain GMO beet sugar, which really isn't much better. It can also contain quite a lot of sugar in some form, so read the full label.

"No sugar added"/"Sugar-free" – Often means that there is artificial sweetener added instead. Check the label and look for 'sucralose' or 'aspartame' on there. *Some* products are only sweetened with fruit juices, but you have to read the ingredients label to know for sure. "Sugar free" is more likely to contain artificial sweeteners.

"All Natural" – This means absolutely nothing. If the food was made from ingredients that, at one point, grew outside, it can be labeled this way (even if the ingredients are highly processed). Cans of processed meals can be labeled this way. Ignore this claim. (This is especially important because one study[113] shows that more people pay attention to 'natural' than 'organic' even though organic is regulated and natural isn't!)

"Good for you!" – Also means nothing. There is no basis or regulation of this claim. The product probably contains synthetic vitamins and minerals, but could also contain a lot of preservatives and other junk.

"Made with real fruit" – The product can contain 1% highly processed fruit juice and make this claim. It does not mean there is any actual, whole fruit in the product at all.

"Pesticide-Free" – This is not a regulated claim. It basically means there's no obvious residue, but it doesn't mean that the product wasn't grown with pesticides. It can still be conventional (and usually is).

"Raw" – Usually applied to cheese, it means that it is heated below the legal point of pasteurization, which is 176. However, most of these cheeses have been heated to around 160 degrees, which is well above the point at which raw enzymes are killed (that's about 120). This is not actually raw, but since it's not technically pasteurized either, it's labeled raw.

"Uncured" – This is applied to meats like bacon, hot dogs, etc. It means that no chemical nitrates were used, but it usually also means that celery juice or another 'natural' source of nitrates were used instead. It is uncertain whether this is any better.

"Contains no _____" – This means that a particular ingredient isn't added (vegetable oil, trans fats, etc.). It does not make the product actually healthy. There are a lot of ingredients that consumers don't usually know to avoid, like modified food starch, which can be found in many products even in health food stores. Also, the serving size may have been adjusted to be unnaturally small, so that each contains less than 0.5g of that ingredient per serving...and may therefore be legally labeled as not containing it. But this does not mean the ingredient wasn't used.

The bottom line? Ignore health claims on the front of the label. They are meaningless. Remember that they are just marketing claims, and not actual claims about how healthy the product is or isn't, over all. They're just intended to play on consumers' desires and to sell them the product...and nothing more.

Read the actual ingredients in the product to see what it contains and if anything jumps out as especially good or bad. See the previous section on ingredients that should be avoided.

---

113   http://articles.mercola.com/sites/articles/archive/2012/12/18/general-mills-cheerios.aspx

KID-FRIENDLY SNACK IDEAS

Kids eat. A lot. If I had a nickel for every time one of my kids said "I'm hungry" or "I want a snack" in a day, I'd be rich! I feel like I do nothing but serve my kids food some days.

Many kids are like this, and the best plan is to have a lot of healthy snack foods on hand. Snacking is *not* bad unless the snack offered is junk. If "snack" is usually chips, pretzels, candy, etc. then snacking is bad. But if "snack" is cheese, fruit, etc. (real foods) then snacking is fine. Children who are offered healthy, whole foods will eat what they need and won't have a problem (see the section on obesity).

Of course, feeding kids all these healthy snacks requires having options on hand! Here are some great kid-friendly healthy snack ideas:

- Whole wheat or gluten-free crackers (preferably homemade) with cheese or nut butter
- Apple slices or celery with nut butter[114]
- Dried fruits (cranberries, raisins, cherries, blueberries, banana chips)
- Jerky[115]
- Chunks of raw cheese
- Plain yogurt (add fruit and/or honey if desired)
- Applesauce
- Home-canned fruits[116], or commercial if packed in 100% juice
- Smoothies[117]
- Popsicles[118] made from yogurt and fruit
- Almond flour muffins[119]
- Coconut flour muffins[120] (coconut + banana[121] is easy and popular)
- Whole wheat soaked muffins (waffles, other breads)
- Fermented veggies (pickles, sauerkraut, dilly carrots, etc.)
- "Meringue" cookies
- Soaked granola bars
- Fresh fruit or veggies, with homemade dips[122] (avoid store-bought; see last section)

---

114   http://www.modernalternativemama.com/blog/2012/10/11/recipe-collection-mixed-nut-butter/ #.ULfKiuRJOAg
115   http://www.modernalternativemama.com/blog/2010/2/8/making-jerky.html
116   http://www.modernalternativemama.com/blog/2012/08/03/my-preserving-plan-and-how-to-can-peaches-without-sugar/
117   http://www.modernalternativemama.com/blog/2010/9/9/recipe-collection-favorite-smoothie.html
118   http://www.modernalternativemama.com/blog/2010/3/25/recipe-collection-fruity-kefir-popsicles. html
119   http://www.modernalternativemama.com/blog/2011/1/20/recipe-collection-almond-flour-muffins. html
120   http://www.modernalternativemama.com/blog/2011/1/20/recipe-collection-almond-flour-muffins. html
121   http://www.modernalternativemama.com/blog/2012/08/02/recipe-collection-banana-muffins/
122   http://www.modernalternativemama.com/store/breast-to-bib/

- Hummus with soaked pitas or veggies
- Milkshakes (raw milk, cream, ice, maple syrup, pastured egg yolks, banana, cocoa powder, etc.)
- Raw fudge (cocoa powder, butter or coconut oil, honey)
- Fresh fruit and vegetable juice (carrot, apple, pineapple, parsley, beet, ginger, blueberry, etc.)
- Whole milk (plain, or mix with maple syrup, cocoa powder, and vanilla for chocolate milk)
- Kefir (mix with strawberries and honey, or any other fruit as desired)
- Soaked nuts[123]
- White bean cake[124]
- Trail mix (homemade)
- Chocolate-hazelnut sauce[125] with crackers, bread, or fruit
- Soaked bread and butter[126]
- Sausage balls[127]
- Guacamole[128] with veggies
- Leftovers from any meal

If you find recipes that work, try making large batches and freezing them. It is easy to make several dozen mini-muffins at once, or can several quarts of fruit, or make big batches of granola bars or trail mix. It doesn't take much longer to make a triple batch rather than a single batch, so do it! Always freeze the extras quickly because if your kids are like mine, they will quickly pounce on and eat anything that they can find.

Having homemade goodness on hand means that snacks will be healthy and easy, at home or on the go!

---

123   http://www.modernalternativemama.com/blog/2011/12/1/recipe-collection-how-to-make-crispy-nuts.html

124   http://www.modernalternativemama.com/blog/2011/12/1/recipe-collection-how-to-make-crispy-nuts.html

125   http://www.modernalternativemama.com/blog/2011/6/16/recipe-collection-chocolate-hazelnut-sauce.html

126   http://www.modernalternativemama.com/blog/2012/04/19/recipe-collection-honey-oat-bread/

127   http://www.modernalternativemama.com/blog/2012/06/07/recipe-collection-sausage-balls/

128   http://www.modernalternativemama.com/blog/2012/02/16/recipe-collection-guacamole/

KID-FRIENDLY LUNCH BOX IDEAS

If your kids go to school, or even if you take lunch "on the go" fairly often for play dates or homeschooling trips, you need lunch box ideas. The standard white-bread-and-pressed-meat sandwich isn't a good idea. So...what do you feed your kids for lunch?

Any of the ideas in the 'snack' section above are also good for lunch, but I do have some additional ideas for you.

- Real meat sandwiches on soaked bread[129] (add veggies, raw cheese, as desired)
- Salads (add meat, crispy nuts, raw cheese, and homemade dressing)
- Hard-boiled eggs (pastured if possible)
- Cold brown rice pasta with tomato or meat sauce
- Chicken and rice
- Leftover soups[130] (anything homemade is great; make your own bone broth)
- Tuna salad (make your own mayo)
- Sausage and potatoes (fry them up together)
- Scrambled eggs (leftover/cold) or omelets
- Pizza balls[131]
- Philly cheesesteak pockets[132]
- Fresh lemonade (for a treat)
- Raw milk

Basically anything leftover is great – soups, salads, sandwiches, pastas are great too. Add some of the snack ideas and you have a health lunch box!

---

129   http://www.modernalternativemama.com/blog/2012/04/19/recipe-collection-honey-oat-bread/
130   http://www.modernalternativemama.com/blog/2012/05/17/recipe-collection-half-a-chicken-soup/
131   http://www.modernalternativemama.com/blog/2012/05/31/recipe-collection-pizza-balls/
132   http://www.modernalternativemama.com/blog/2012/06/28/recipe-collection-philly-cheesesteak-pockets/

KID-FRIENDLY FOOD ON A BUDGET

A big concern for many parents is how to feed their children well on a budget. Although many of us would like to prioritize food and spend "whatever it takes" to get healthy food into our children, that is not the reality that we face when we look at the budget. We are limited by the amount of money we have available. For some families this is more than others, depending on their personal finances, and a few families would be able to move some funds from "discretionary" areas to the food budget if needed. Other families have cut everything possible and still do not have as much in their food budget as they'd like. What then?

Choose Cheap Food Items

A lot of what we buy is brown rice, potatoes, carrots, celery, wheat berries, and other fairly common, inexpensive foods (these are all purchased organic because they are not any more expensive in our area than conventional). Other cheap food items include peas, broccoli, onions, garlic, squash, oats, barley, beans, bananas, and so on (not organic for us). Focus meals around these items; they contain plenty of nutrition. Make soups and stews, especially for kids who won't eat the veggies on their own.

Prioritize Organic

Buy only items on the dirty dozen list organically, as well as animal products where possible (here, prioritize the ones you buy most often if you can't afford all). It is not necessary to buy *everything* organic. Those dirty dozen items that are simply expensive organically (berries tend to be, as well as grapes) can be rare purchases. We love them too, but I can't afford $4/lb. with the way my kids eat grapes.

Grow Your Own

If you have the space and time, try growing your own. Even those with limited space can start with a few potted herbs. Those with larger space can plant extensive gardens and grow most of their own food. Grow what you are most likely to eat and especially those items that are more expensive in your area, if possible. You can completely control what goes into/onto the plants. Buy yourself a good organic gardening guide and read it cover to cover several times if you're new to gardening before beginning; it will strongly increase your yields and decrease frustration.

Look for Local Farms

The prices directly from local farms is going to be a lot better than buying the same items in a health food store – and the quality will probably be higher. Grass-fed (but not finished) ground beef at Whole Foods in my area is $6/lb. From a local butcher, I can get completely grass-fed beef for $2.29/lb. when I buy in bulk (and farms usually run around $4.50/lb.). Eggs that are "okay" would be around $4 - $5/doz. at a health food store; they're $2.50/doz from a farm. Find local farms in your area for the best prices and quality whenever possible. Check www.eatwild.com or ask around for more information; farms can be hard to find at first (I once had *no* clue where to even start and now I know dozens of farms). Once you get 'in the network' so to speak, you'll find a lot more. One word of caution: farmer's markets are often not the best place to buy because they tend to be as expensive or more so than grocery stores in many areas. Visit them just to get to know local farms and then contact them individually to ask for bulk prices (see below).

Buy Seasonal and Stock Up

We love blueberries, but out of season, they're $5/lb. – for frozen (and a lot more for fresh). In season we can pick at a local organic blueberry patch for $2.50/lb. I borrow all the adults I can find to help pick and watch children and go pick a ton. When apples are $0.50/lb. because they're in season, I buy a whole bunch. We eat them fresh, and we preserve them. When tomatoes are in season they're as cheap as apples and we also buy a lot of those. It's also true that what is cheap in each area varies, so take advantage of what is cheap in your area. I have friends who can get blueberries for $1/lb. or less in other states. On the coast, fresh seafood is very cheap. Look for what's bountiful in your area and focus on that. Enjoy the bounty while you can.

Preserve Your Own

When I said we buy *a lot*, I meant it. In fall 2012 we did over 400 lbs. of tomatoes and around 160 lbs. of apples (which wasn't nearly as much as I'd wanted; I'd have done 400+ lbs. of those if I'd been able to get them). These were turned into applesauce, fruit leather, and apple pie filling. Tomatoes were turned into diced tomatoes, tomato sauce, tomato soup, and salsa. I will freeze 40 – 50 lbs. each of strawberries and blueberries (blueberries are a bit more expensive but our family prefers them). Zucchini is shredded and frozen for adding to breads, soups, etc. later. Learn to freeze what you can and try out canning – it is such a great way to access very high quality food for a fraction of the price. We've recently gotten a pressure canner so that we can do vegetables and meats (including stock) as well!

No Packaged Foods

It is rare that I spend more than $10 of grocery money every couple of weeks on anything in a package, for budget reasons more than anything else. Healthy premade snacks are expensive, and so are healthier "ingredients," like tortillas, sandwich bread, etc. If you can avoid them, do so – make your own versions instead. There are several excellent cookbooks out there to teach you how to replace snacks, breads, condiments, and other expensive items with homemade, healthier, cheaper versions.

Shop Discount and Warehouse Stores

Costco and even places like Aldi or "scratch'n'dent" type grocery stores can sometimes have good options. Look for places in your area and buy what you can there. I look around Amish Country a few times a year for options like these and also head to cheaper stores when I can. Buy in bulk where possible, especially if you do prefer a few convenience items for whatever reason (they have freeze-dried fruit snacks at Costco that we buy from time to time). There is no shame in shopping at Walmart, either, if that is what you can afford. There is no sense in paying more for the same product when your grocery budget is already stretched.

Coop with Friends

Many online stores offer great prices and often free shipping if you order in bulk. Ordering by yourself is not always possible, of course (laying out $150 at once is a lot!). Get some friends to go in on the items with you and order in bulk that way. We have done this with cheese, coconut oil, FCLO, nuts, and a number of other products. (See the resources at the end of this section.)

Use Kitchen Scraps

Potato peels can be brushed with butter and salt and baked. Fruit pulp from juicing can be dried as a fruit bar. Extra egg whites can be whipped into meringue cookies (recipe in this book). Lemon peels can be dried for herbal tea. Bones can (should!) be used to make stock for soups and stews. Fruit cores and other fruit/vegetable scraps can be juiced (pineapple cores in particular are really rich in bromelain, a potent antioxidant). See what you can make use of, even if it's not something you would normally eat. Somewhat sour (raw) milk can be used to bake or mixed with fruit and honey for popsicles. This is a big way that I get snacks for my kids!

No Waste

To go along with the last one, don't waste food. Some 30% of the food the average family buys is wasted! Use leftovers quickly or freeze them. Turn leftovers into other meals if you like – leftover meat into soups or mix with eggs. Go through your vegetable drawer at least weekly and make a plan to use up whatever is there, even if it just means chopping and freezing for another day. Check through the pantry for odds and ends. A small amount of beans or pasta or rice can be tossed into any sort of soup. Label your leftovers and consider writing a list of them on a dry erase board on your fridge if you're likely to forget they are there until it's too late.

Stretch the Meat

Add beans, make soups, don't serve meat as the center of the meal. If you do serve meat as the main meal, try breading it and frying in a healthy oil like coconut oil, or adding homemade bread crumbs, eggs, and veggies and turning it into meatloaf. Choose to make meatless meals. A lot of meatless meals (like soups) can be made with bone broth so they're still nutrient-rich.

Soak the Grains

Soaked grains make them more digestible and more nutritious. They're more filling. We especially like soaked waffles, which are rich in whole grains, raw milk, and eggs. They're fairly cheap to make and great for quick breakfasts or snacks. Soaked rice or barley can go into soups and stews to increase nutrition and make them more filling as well.

Add Fat

Don't be afraid of fat. Add extra butter to anything. Drizzle olive oil over pasta or salads or even meat just prior to serving (don't heat it if possible). Olive oil mixed with herbs is also great for dipping bread into. (Try the soaked no-knead bread in this book.) Pan-fry meat and fish with some coconut oil, beef tallow, or lard. Make "candy" from coconut oil, honey, shredded coconut, and chocolate (if you like).

Buy What You Can

If what you can afford is real grocery store cheese from a discount store (not processed cheese, but not grass-fed or hormone/antibiotic free), then buy that. If what you can afford is real meat from a grocery store, buy that. It is better to buy plain ingredients, whatever their quality, and cook than it is to buy processed foods with all kinds of additives. Be picky if you have the resources to be able to do so; but if not, don't feel guilty about buying what you can afford. Unprocessed foods will always be better than processed no matter where they come from.

When you're on a budget, you have to be creative. Do what you can, use everything you have, take any gift of free food (like when your neighbor has an overflowing garden in the summer!), and call it good.

Resources:

www.farmcountrycheese.com (grass-fed cheeses for good prices)

www.wildernessfamilynaturals.com (lots of pantry items; we especially buy the coconut products. Best quality and best prices.)

www.homegrownalmonds.com (good prices on natural almonds)

www.azurestandard.com (online bulk ordering for pantry goods; drop points in some areas)

www.greenpasture.org (fermented cod liver oil; there are buying group accounts available that receive around 20% off 12 bottles or more)

GETTING KIDS INVOLVED IN THE KITCHEN

One of the best ways to get kids on board with healthy eating is to get them involved in the kitchen! It will teach them an important life skill – cooking – as well as the art of traditional, real food preparation. My kids know exactly how to brew kombucha, make stock, soak dough and produce a variety of baked goods by hand, and lots more. If they want lemonade, they head to the fridge to grab a lemon. All of these amazing, healthy foods that I've had to learn to cook as an adult are no big deal to them – they will grow up having been surrounded by it and having helped prepare it from such a young age that it will be second nature to them.

Plus, kids like to help. Whatever Mommy or Daddy is doing is completely fascinating! And there are a lot of ways even small children *can* help in the kitchen! Try some of these:

- Dumping in pre-measured ingredients (muffins, etc.)
- Stirring bowls
- Kneading dough (very small ones, under 2, will eat it – but unless it contains raw factory eggs or something that's okay)
- Rolling out dough
- Peeling vegetables (from age 4 or 5)
- Chopping vegetables (sometimes 4 – 5 year-olds can do this)
- Cracking eggs
- Finding ingredients
- Putting ingredients away
- Putting baked goods into a cold oven (if it doesn't need preheating)
- Stirring at the stove (from age 6 or 7)
- Making waffles (using the iron alone – from age 7 or 8)

There are a lot of ways to help! The very small ones can be given a little bit of ingredients to "play" with even while you are in the kitchen – a small amount of flour, water, whatever you have. Older kids can start to take on more tasks and by the time they are 8 or so, can even cook meals by themselves. The more they help when they are small, the more they will be independent in the kitchen at a young age.

This is great for both boys and girls, because everyone needs the basic life skill of cooking. Starting them young means they'll be forever comfortable in the kitchen!

KID-FRIENDLY RECIPES

Feeding kids healthy foods can be easier said than done. We, as adults, know what they "should" eat, but they may or may not agree to actually eat it!

That's why I've included a small handful of healthy, kid-friendly recipes in this book. It's not primarily a cookbook, but these recipes will get you started with some healthier options for your kids. You'll find our favorite cookies, breakfast waffles, and even a super-healthy version of spaghetti sauce!

If you need more inspiration, see our other books (which are all cookbooks):

Real Food Basics – Real food versions of family-favorites: tomato sauce, meatloaf, coffee cake, French fries, pizza dough, and more.

Healthy Pregnancy Super Foods – Super-food based recipes (good for everyone, not just pregnant women!): chicken and wild rice soup, Italian wedding soup, pork chops and rice, salmon with garlic-herb butter, chicken marsala, refried beans, mozzarella sticks, maple cinnamon granola bars, and more.

Against the Grain – A book for those on low-grain or grain-free diets (or gluten-free), including GAPS: Sausage with peppers and spaghetti squash, fish in white sauce, Salisbury steak, beef tips with Portobello mushrooms, tomato-cream sauce with chicken and zucchini, sausage gumbo, Italian chili, white bean vanilla cake, chocolate chip bread, and more.

Treat Yourself: Real Food Desserts – Have your cake and eat it too, with desserts based on nourishing ingredients: cinnamon rolls, strawberry yum-yum, spice cake, lemon cake, chocolate cake, cream cheese frosting, butter cookies, strawberry-peach frozen yogurt, chocolate éclairs, and more.

Wholesome Comfort – Comfort food without the canned soups and processed cheese: roast beef, chicken pot pie, chicken and dumplings, cream soup base, twice-baked potatoes, breakfast sausage, Italian chicken, scalloped potatoes, green bean casserole, pumpkin spice ice cream, chocolate fudge, and more.

Breast to Bib – A book filled with toddler and kid-friendly recipes (as well as information on how to best feed the littlest ones): chicken nuggets, popcorn chicken, quesadillas, barbecue sauce, honey-mustard sauce, guacamole, chocolate pudding, pigs in a blanket, cheese sauce, peanut butter chocolate chip granola bars, chocolate hazelnut balls, and more.

Simply Summer – Summer-inspired recipes using seasonal and local ingredients: tomato and cucumber salad, grilled shrimp salad, bacon-cheddar dip, tropical punch, bacon-wrapped chicken with Italian salsa, bacon spinach and tomato pasta, pita chips, fruit salad with poppy seed dressing, roasted garlic vinaigrette, peach upside down cake, lemon sherbet, salty caramel ice cream, and more!

Festive Traditions – A holiday-inspired collection of real food favorites: spinach-artichoke dip, autumn stuffed squash, butternut squash soup with ginger cream, stuffed mushrooms, egg nog, bacon-wrapped dates, buckeyes, apple cake with caramel sauce, and more.

Choose one or more that work for your family – all can be found at www.

SOAKED GRANOLA BARS

My kids love granola bars, but they don't so well with unsoaked oats – which means we have to make our own. These worked out really well and were a hit with the kids! They're a very basic recipe, so feel free to mix up the flavors or add some "additions" to the bars if you like.

Ingredients:

4 c. rolled oats

1 c. whole wheat flour or buckwheat flour (for gluten-free)

10 tbsp. butter, softened (or coconut oil)

¾ c. raw honey

1 tsp. vanilla

1 tsp. cinnamon*

1 tsp. sea salt

*May leave out if you prefer, especially if adding extra ingredients

Directions:

At night, mix together the oats, wheat or buckwheat flour, butter or coconut oil, and raw honey. Cover this and allow it to sit overnight.

In the morning, add the vanilla, cinnamon, and sea salt. Stir to combine thoroughly, then press the mixture into a 9x13 baking pan. Bake at 350 for about 25 – 30 minutes, until the edges are golden brown. Remove from the oven and allow them to cool. They will fall apart if sliced while they are still hot; they do much better if they are cooled before slicing.

Additions:

*1/2 c. mini chocolate chips

*1/2 c. shredded coconut

*1/2 c. chopped crispy nuts (almonds, walnuts, etc.)

*1/2 c. dried fruit (raisins, cranberries, etc.)

Add 1 – 2 additions, no more than 1 c. total. Feel free to add extra vanilla or try a little ground ginger, cloves, etc. for other "spice" varieties.

Makes 10 – 12 servings.

Serving Suggestion:
Pair with a fruit smoothie for a quick and healthy breakfast.

"MERINGUE" COOKIES

These are one of my kids' favorite treats, yet they are very healthy, low-sugar, and high in protein. They also use up extra egg whites (which we always seem to have a lot of). A few egg whites makes a very big batch of these so they are easy to have around for snacks.

Ingredients:

4 egg whites
2 tbsp. raw honey or grade B maple syrup
1 tsp. vanilla
1 tbsp. cocoa powder (optional)

Directions:

Add all the ingredients to a large glass bowl. Use a mixer to whip the egg whites until soft and fluffy and stiff peaks form.

Scoop the cookies onto parchment-paper lined cookie sheets. Bake at 350 for 10 – 12 minutes, until golden brown. Serve as-is, or turn the oven off and allow them to dry for a few hours so they are crunchy. If making several batches at once, the parchment paper sheets can also go into a dehydrator to dry overnight.

Store in an air-tight container for a few days.

Makes 3 – 4 dozen.

Serving Suggestion:
Pair with some herbal tea for a quick snack.

SURPRISE SPAGHETTI SAUCE

This is one of my favorites, and most kids who enjoy spaghetti will love it too – and they'll never know what's in it!

Ingredients:

1 lb. ground beef

¼ lb. liver, rinsed well and chopped into tiny pieces

1 small onion, minced

2 – 3 garlic cloves, minced

1 small zucchini, shredded

4 c. tomato sauce (preferably homemade) or puree

2 c. beef stock

2 tsp. basil

1 tsp. oregano

1 tsp. sea salt, or to taste

Directions:

Saute the ground beef and liver with the onion and garlic in a large saucepan until the meat is done. Add the remaining ingredients (adjusting the spices up or down depending on if you are using puree or sauce with spices already added). Simmer for an hour or two. The "extras" will not even be noticeable once the sauce is done! Serve over brown rice pasta.

If desired, add up to 2 c. chopped veggies (zucchini, mushrooms, bell peppers, etc.) to the sauce when sautéing the meat and veggies.

Makes 8 – 10 servings.

Serving Suggestion:

Pour on top of spaghetti squash or brown rice pasta for a healthy meal any time.

SOAKED WAFFLES

This is one of our favorites and I often make up a quadruple batch at once! It takes a few hours one morning to bake them all, but then they're in the freezer for a couple weeks and breakfast takes only a couple minutes to get on the table. They also make good snacks at other times of day. Top with butter, a little real maple syrup, real whipped cream and fruit, or whatever you like for a healthy and filling meal.

Ingredients:

3 c. freshly ground whole wheat flour

½ c. butter, melted or softened

2 – 3 c. raw milk, divided

2 eggs

3 tbsp. maple syrup or sucanat

2 tsp. sea salt

1 tbsp. baking powder

1 tsp. vanilla

Directions:

At night, mix together the flour, butter, and enough milk to make a very soft dough or thick batter (about 2 c.). Cover and allow it to sit for about 12 hours. (Longer is okay but it will get increasingly sour.)

In the morning, add 1 c. milk, eggs, sucanat, sea salt, baking powder, and vanilla to the blender. Begin blending until the liquid ingredients are well incorporated. While the blender is running on low, add the soaked batter until it is completely smooth and fairly thick.

Pour into a pre-heated waffle iron and bake according to device directions, until done. Repeat with remaining batter.

Serve immediately, or allow the waffles to cool before freezing. If frozen, toast before serving.

Makes about 12 waffles.

Serving Suggestion:

Top with butter and serve with fresh fruit or bacon for a quick, healthy breakfast.

SOAKED NO-KNEAD BREAD

The idea behind no-knead bread is simple: combine yeast, salt, flour, and water, stir together to form a soft dough, then let it rise and bake without having to knead at all. Simple! But how can you do it in a soaked form? I created this version and it works. And it's yummy. Serve it with olive oil dip, butter, or use it for sandwiches!

Ingredients:

4 c. white whole wheat flour, freshly ground

½ c. olive oil

2 c. warm water

2 tsp. sea salt

3 tsp. yeast

Directions:

Combine flour, oil, and water in a large glass bowl. Stir until a soft dough forms. Let this sit in a warm place overnight. In the morning, sprinkle sea salt and yeast over the dough and knead/stir very briefly, just long enough to incorporate it. Pick it up and stretch it, fold it for about a minute until mixed. Cover and allow it to sit in a warm place until doubled, 1 – 2 hours.

Pour the dough onto an ungreased baking sheet. Bake at 450 for 15 minutes, then an additional 15 – 20 minutes at 400. The edges should be golden brown. Wait until it is cool to slice. If you slice while hot, the texture may be weird and the bread may not seem done – but it is.

Makes 8 – 10 servings.

Serving Suggestion:

Dip in olive oil or slather with butter for a quick snack.

SECTION 2: HEALTH

WHAT DOES IT MEAN TO BE "HEALTHY?"

These days, it's hard to know what "health" really is. For some, it's a lack of chronic conditions. For others, it means chronic conditions are well-managed. Most people consider themselves healthy as long as they are able to function day-to-day in most respects.

This is a sad definition of "health."

Many people still suffer from allergies, asthma, attention disorders, gut imbalances, diabetes, obesity, and many other conditions. This is not *health*! Ideally, we want to avoid these conditions entirely. That is not always possible, for one reason or another – genetics, approaching a healthier lifestyle later in the game, and so on. But we need to understand that these things aren't *normal* and that really healthy people don't have them.

Parents have come to believe the following conditions are "normal" (as in, many people have them and there's nothing that can be done) when, in fact, they are not:

- Colic
- Eczema
- Asthma
- Diabetes
- Allergies (food/environmental)
- ADHD
- Autism
- Learning disabilities
- Picky eating

We *can* do something about many of these, in many cases. Not for all, but for many. There are things that influence a child's health before s/he is born as well as after. The mother's health, vitamin D status, breastfeeding, first foods, environmental situations (see the next section) and so on all influence a child's health. You can read about many of the new baby and young toddler health issues in my book *Breast to Bib*.

True health is about an absence of "conditions" where at all possible. It's about optimal gut health. It's about *feeling good* most of the time – not just 'not bad,' but actually *good*. I did not know the difference myself until I switched to real food! Now it is very obvious.

Watching children it is obvious too. Children who don't feel well are more likely to feel lethargic and want to sit around, have trouble concentrating, or be irritable. Children who do feel well want to run, play, laugh, and have fun! They have boundless energy. True health strives for the latter.

While this is what we are talking about when we say "real health," that doesn't mean that if you are new coming into this and your child already has some health concerns that your child can't be healthy. It doesn't mean that children with chronic or genetic conditions can't be healthy. Their definition of health is a bit different, but they can still be healthier than they would otherwise be if they eat well and focus on simple health solutions where possible.

Of course, if your child *does* have specific health needs, talk to your doctor before taking any of the advice in this book. The dietary and home remedy information is meant for healthy children without chronic conditions and in self-limiting, acute cases. Children whose health requires managing need to seek appropriate medical care. (And I do encourage finding an alternatively-minded doctor if at all possible, so that s/he can guide you as to what tests/treatments are truly necessary and which natural options you may be able to use also.)

WELL-CHILD VISITS: SHOULD YOU?

One of the typical cornerstones of early childhood health is the well-child visit. But... should you? Do you have to?

There are arguments on both sides. Let's examine this further.

The Case for Well-Child Visits

One of the primary purposes of well-child visits is vaccinating. Children who follow the CDC schedule[133] receive vaccines at their 2, 4, 6, 12, 15, 18, and 24-month visits (as well as 4 or 5 years, 11 – 12 years, and perhaps immediately before college, as well as annual flu shots). This coincides exactly with the typical well-child visit schedule. If you do plan to follow the CDC vaccine schedule, then you will need to attend all the visits.

Another reason for well-child visits is to develop a relationship with a doctor. If a concern about a child's health ever arises, the doctor will be familiar with the child's medical history and able to address the concern more accurately than a doctor who is not familiar with the child.

In some cases, pediatricians can catch certain developmental or other health concerns early, simply by seeing the child regularly. Screening questions or tests can turn up a concern and allow parents to receive an early diagnosis and early intervention, if needed. Pediatricians are more aware of what to look for in these areas than parents are, especially first-time parents.

Having a record of well-child visits also protects parents, especially those who choose to follow an alternative lifestyle, from being accused of medical neglect. An ongoing record showing regular well-child visits goes a long way to negate such accusations, supposing they are ever made.

There are many reasons, obviously, for choosing to do well-child visits. But there are also plenty of reasons not to.

The Case Against Well-Child Visits

Not all parents follow the CDC vaccine schedule. Some follow an alternative/delayed schedule[134], and some choose to forgo vaccines all together. For parents who do not vaccinate or who delay until after age 1 or 2, taking the baby to the doctor every couple of months may seem like overkill – especially if they are not first-time parents. These parents may choose to skip some or all of the well-child check ups.

Every time a child goes into a doctor's office, s/he has the potential to be exposed to illness – just by the nature of what doctors do. Even with careful hygiene and separate waiting areas (which not all doctors have), children are at greater risk of catching something in a doctor's office than almost any other place. Some parents do not feel that the risk to their child of getting sick is worth the benefit of the visit. After all, if the doctor is primarily going to weigh and measure the child, that is nothing that the parents can't do at home.

There is also the fact that for a variety of reasons, most doctors cannot spend more than

---

133   http://www.cdc.gov/vaccines/schedules/
134   http://www.askdrsears.com/topics/vaccines/alternative-vaccine-schedule

5 – 10 minutes[135] with their patients. Even the excellent ones can only carve out 30 – 40 minutes for each patient. Seeing patients for this short amount of time every few months to annually is not enough time to really "know" or be familiar with a patient. A parent who does truly know their child would be more likely to notice if something were "off" with that child sooner than a doctor would for this very reason. Doctors also may refer patients or not based on inherent biases and not take parental concerns seriously[136].

(Which is a good reason to have a doctor with whom you have an excellent partnership, and one whom you trust. Then if something ever did seem to be wrong, the doctor would listen carefully to the parent's observations and instincts and treat the child in conjunction with the parents.)

In some cases, doctor choice is limited and parents are forced to see doctors who do not respect their wishes, who are quick to prescribe drugs[137], or who offer bad, outdated medical advice (such as offering solids to a two-week-old baby). In these cases, the frustration of dealing with a doctor who is unhelpful may outweigh any benefits of having a relationship with a doctor.

Pediatricians, while experts in children's health, disease, and treating growing and developing children, are not often experts in practical matters that parents really need help with – breastfeeding[138], carseat safety, helping babies to sleep, and so on. Pediatricians are often even less helpful with 'alternative' parents, as they do not know much about and may actively recommend against extended breastfeeding, extended rear-facing in the car, co-sleeping, and other common alternative practices.

The Bottom Line

No one can decide if you should do well-child visits except for you. If you are vaccinating or if your child has a particular health concern, you will probably choose to do them. If your child does not have any particular health concerns and/or if you have chosen to take your child through an alternative care route, you may opt not to do well-child visits.

Personally we took our first two children to nearly all the usual well-child visits (skipping only my second's 15-month visit as we were in the process of changing doctors). Our third has seen a doctor only twice, at 6 weeks and 6 months, and it is uncertain if our fourth will see a doctor at all, unless there is a concern.

Our children do see a chiropractor weekly, and we do usually take the kids for annual visits with the pediatrician – but by no means do we feel we need all the usual visits. On the few occasions our children have been sick enough to warrant a call to the doctor (once each for our oldest two and never for our youngest), the chiropractor was our first stop and another local alternative doctor was our second.

Many other parents choose a similar route – having a chiropractor or another 'alternative' doctor as their primary care physician. See the section on Alternative Doctors for more about this.

Talk it over with your husband or significant other and make a decision based on your

135   http://healthland.time.com/2011/09/19/one-third-of-pediatricians-breeze-in-and-out-yet-parents-seem-satisfied/
136   http://pediatrics.aappublications.org/content/113/2/274.abstract
137   http://www.sciencedaily.com/releases/2007/07/070726091218.htm
138   http://pediatrics.aappublications.org/content/103/3/e35.full

family's needs. Remember it is your choice and you don't have to do some, all, or none just because that's what others have chosen. Every family will do things differently and that is okay.

A NOTE ON VACCINES

Over the last 15 years or so, vaccines have become increasingly controversial. There are parents who would never consider going without the full CDC schedule, and parents who would never consider injecting their children with such "poison." There are parents who choose a middle ground, doing only selected vaccines or choosing to delay or space them out.

New parents who are approaching this issue quickly find it is a thorny one. There is not a lot of solid science on either side yet; although there is emerging science to support a variety of positions. It also tends to be an extremely emotional, hot-button issue for many families. A lot of parents have chosen, at least in part, to vaccinate or not because they know someone who was seriously ill with a vaccine-preventable disease or because they know someone who was injured by a vaccine. Parents who are looking for unemotional, science-based information are hard-pressed to find it.

This is a really sad state because parents deserve access to unbiased, scientific information when they are making such an important decision for their children. Vaccination, like any medical decision, should not be an emotional one, but a fact-based one.

Despite what parents have been told by doctors and the mainstream media, there *is* science to suggest that vaccines are linked to ADHD[139], autism, asthma, and a number of other serious chronic conditions. In no way have these questions been settled, and in no way has a vaccine-autism link been debunked, as is often stated. (In no way has it been fully proven, either; nor are vaccines the only factor in autism. There are many, many factors, largely environmental in nature.)

At the end of November, 2012, there was a congressional hearing[140]. This hearing was not covered by the mainstream media whatsoever; it did air live on C-SPAN 3, for those who get the channel. The upshot was that expert after expert testified that vaccines are associated with chronic and degenerative disease and plenty of parents told their stories as well. The leaders of the CDC and the NIH were called, and could not answer any questions. They could not provide any data to support the idea that vaccines weren't responsible for chronic illness or anything else. They could not point to any studies that had been done or which were currently in progress that accurately studied the difference between vaccinated and unvaccinated children. Official sources are starting to recognize that the evidence proving that vaccines are safe isn't there.

It is important for parents to understand that the debate has *not* been settled and there is no obvious answer. This book and this section are not intended to convince parents one way or another, but to open up the idea that it is necessary to ask questions and not accept "what most people say."

Questions parents should ask:

- What are the ingredients in vaccines?[141]
- How serious are these diseases?

---

139   http://fourteenstudies.org/ourstudies.html
140   http://thinkingmomsrevolution.com/great-what-now/
141   http://www.cdc.gov/vaccines/pubs/pinkbook/downloads/appendices/B/excipient-table-2.pdf

- What is the likelihood of catching each disease?
- What is the likelihood of developing complications from each?
- What is the likelihood of serious/permanent issues or death from each disease?
- Is there any long-term benefit to any of these diseases?
- What is the likelihood of a vaccine reaction?[142]
- What is the likelihood of a severe vaccine reaction?
- Is the benefit of the vaccine worth the risk?

It is unfortunately very hard to answer these questions. There is very little unbiased science out there. It is important for parents to know that when new vaccines are being studied for reactions, the "placebo" used is not a true placebo[143] – it is a previously licensed version of the vaccine or a combination of all the vaccine ingredients minus the antigen. A true placebo would be saline, something with no chemicals whatsoever. It is true that sometimes researchers "throw out" data[144] that doesn't fit their general data set (including the rare severe reactions).

Reading vaccine package inserts[145] is a great place to start. Although not unbiased, they are more accurate than many of the "fact sheets" passed out by the CDC or doctors' offices. Another good resource is the CDC's "Pink Book[146]," which is the fact book intended for medical professionals. It is a lot more accurate and science-based than the fact sheets intended for parents.

There are several other good resources out there:

- *The Vaccine Book*, by Dr. Robert Sears
- *Vaccinations: The Thoughtful Parent's Guide: How to Make Safe, Sensible Decisions about the Risks, Benefits and Alternatives*, by Aviva Jill Romm, M.D.
- *Callous Disregard: Autism and Vaccines: The Truth Behind the Tragedy*, by Dr. Andrew J. Wakefield
- *Make an Informed Vaccine Decision for the Health of Your Child: A Guide to Childhood Shots*, by Dr. Mayer Eisenstein
- *Vaccines: Are They Really Safe and Effective*, by Neil Z. Miller
- *How to Raise a Health Child in Spite of Your Doctor*, by Dr. Robert S. Mendelsohn
- *What Your Doctor May Not Tell You About Children's Vaccinations*, by Dr. Stephanie Cave

Read through these resources, talk to several different doctors (each doctors has his/her own opinion on vaccines and you cannot trust just one person's opinion – make sure to ask several), and make the decision that is best for your family. Thoroughly investigate vaccines and diseases before making any decision. It is possible to delay until later; it is not possible to take back vaccines that have already been given. It is also true that there are ways besides vaccines to protect your child's health, a major issue that is often ignored. There is more on natural immune-boosting in later sections of this book.

---

142   http://wonder.cdc.gov/vaers.html
143   http://wonder.cdc.gov/vaers.html
144   http://pareonline.net/getvn.asp?v=9&n=6
145   http://www.immunize.org/packageinserts/
146   http://www.cdc.gov/vaccines/pubs/pinkbook/index.html#chapters

Are Vaccines Needed for School?

One reason that some parents choose to vaccinate is because they believe that vaccines are required for their children to go to school. They do not want to break any rules, and so even if they have some personal hesitations, they go ahead and get the vaccines in order to comply with the law.

However, vaccines are *not* required to go to school!

In 48 states (except West Virginia and Mississipi), there are religious and/or philosophical exemptions to vaccines. In all 50 states, there are medical exemptions. In some states, they are harder to get than in others, but they are available. Most states and school districts will not mention these exemptions; they will say that vaccines are required to get into school.

In some cases, employees (like secretaries, teachers, principals) may not know the law and may not know these exemptions are available. In other cases, they do not mention them because they don't really want parents to opt out.

These exemptions can be used for either fully unvaccinated children or partially unvaccinated children. Parents can pick and choose which vaccines they would like their children to receive and when, based on their own research and conversations with their doctors. The school should have nothing to do with it. Parents can check out their state's laws[147] to learn more.

It should also be noted that the legal climate varies from state to state. In some states (especially those with all three exemption options), it is considered false reporting to call children's services for the sole reason that a family does not vaccinate. In other states it is taken seriously and the family may be investigated, but legally the family does have rights and should contact a lawyer if needed. It is unfortunate that this even needs to be mentioned, but parental rights are unfortunately not always respected as they should be.

Our Decision

This is strictly *our decision* and is not intended to sway you one way or another. We have chosen not to get any vaccines for our children – ever. After extensive research (hundreds of hours poring over medical journals, books, talking to a variety of doctors, and so on), we feel that vaccines are potentially very dangerous and that there is too little that we understand about the development of the immune system. Vaccines appear to promote inflammation[148] and high T-cell levels (titres), which new research shows are not associated with permanent immunity[149]. There is some evidence that vaccines may increase the risk of hospitalization and death in infants[150].

In contrast, when children undergo natural infection, they acquire permanent immunity, as well as protection against more serious/chronic infections and even against cancer[151],[152] in some cases. Little is understood yet about the role of healthy gut flora in

---

147   http://www.nvic.org/Vaccine-Laws/state-vaccine-requirements.aspx
148   http://www.devdelay.org/newsletter/articles/pdf/404-vaccines-viruses-and-brain-inflammation.pdf
149   http://vaclib.org/basic/titers-immunity.htm
150   http://vaclib.org/basic/titers-immunity.htm
151   http://www.ncbi.nlm.nih.gov/pmc/articles/PMC2737678/
152   http://www.ncbi.nlm.nih.gov/pubmed/20559706

the development of the immune system[153],[154],[155],[156],[157] but scientists are beginning to believe that it plays a very strong and important role. It is unknown how vaccines affect the development of gut flora, or what relationship there is between vaccines and gut flora[158].

Instead of vaccinating, we choose to protect our children with fermented cod liver oil (low vitamin A[159],[160] and vitamin D[161],[162] levels are associated with increased risk of a number of illnesses, from colds to cancer, as well as increased risk of complications from these illnesses), healthy food (again avoiding deficiencies) and occasional herbal supplements or topical magnesium[163],[164], if needed. We believe that by avoiding deficiencies and not overloading their systems with toxic chemicals from food additives or drugs that they are more likely to fight off illnesses without complication.

So far this has proven to be true. Our children have had their share of colds and the occasional stomach virus, but they typically bounce back in a matter of hours (average length of illness in our children is between 2 and 12 hours) and none have ever required antibiotics. They have never had strep throat, bronchitis, or more serious illnesses. This is not to say it could not happen or that, to some extent, we haven't been lucky. Our oldest is only 5. However, our kids have been far healthier in their early years than we, their parents, were as small children. There's something to be said for that.

Please make sure that you do not make any decisions based on one person's story – ours or anyone else's. This is a huge decision that requires a lot of research, thought, and prayer. It is not a decision we made lightly or that we would want anyone else to make lightly.

If you do ultimately choose a selective/delayed/no vaccine schedule for your family, read on for some alternate ways to treat common childhood conditions, as well as how to boost a child's immune system. Even if you choose to vaccinate, these alternatives can be valuable information. The decision to vaccinate or not is not one that should be taken lightly. Parents who choose not to vaccinate need to remember that it is up to them to boost their child's immune system naturally and to learn about alternative ways to keep their child healthy and recover from any illness they do experience.

Continue to ask, read, research, pray, and do whatever you need to do before coming to the right decision for your family. Also, please remember that no part of this book is medical advice and that any concerns you have should be taken to your family's doctor.

153   http://www.medscape.com/viewarticle/448473_4
154   http://www.sciencedaily.com/releases/2011/05/110525105836.htm
155   http://www.sciencedaily.com/releases/2011/05/110525105836.htm
156   http://www.ncbi.nlm.nih.gov/pubmed/3443432
157   http://www.nytimes.com/2011/04/21/science/21gut.html?_r=0
158   http://www.ncbi.nlm.nih.gov/pmc/articles/PMC3219679/
159   http://summaries.cochrane.org/CD001479/vitamin-a-for-measles-in-children
160   http://pediatrics.aappublications.org/content/91/5/1014.abstract
161   http://www.ncbi.nlm.nih.gov/pmc/articles/PMC2798112/
162   http://children.webmd.com/news/20120806/vitamin-d-deficiency-common-sick-kids
163   http://ods.od.nih.gov/factsheets/Magnesium-HealthProfessional/
164   http://lpi.oregonstate.edu/infocenter/minerals/magnesium/

A NOTE ON OTC MEDICATIONS

These days, most parents are advised to stock their medicine cabinets before their babies even arrive, and to make sure they keep certain "basics" on hand. These basics are considered necessary "just in case" to help sick children.

Nobody wants a sick child to suffer! But are the common OTC medications really as safe and beneficial as they are said to be? Let's take a look at them.

Tylenol

This is an "all purpose" drug, acetaminophen, which is used to reduce fevers and pain in babies and children. It is, however, the leading cause of calls to poison control, and is responsible for thousands of hospital visits annually. It is the leading cause of liver failure, accountable for about half of all cases[165]. Tylenol also depletes glutathione, an amino acid and antioxidant needed for immune function[166]. Its use in infancy also is linked to the later development of asthma[167]. There are safer ways to relieve pain, if needed (see home remedies section) and fevers often do not need to be reduced[168].

Simethicone (Mylicon)

This drug is recommended to relieve pain due to excess gas and is most often suggested for newborns who seem to be in pain or who may be colicky. It is not, however, effective for this use[169]. (In fact, the safer and more overall beneficial probiotics were shown to be significantly more effective[170].) There are no well-studied side effects to this drug; however, with safer and more effective alternatives, it does not need to be in the medicine cabinet.

Benadryl

This is an antihistamine that is commonly used to stop allergic reactions as well as to induce drowsiness in certain cases. It has side effects like drowsiness, dizziness, constipation, stomach upset, blurred vision, or dry mouth/nose[171]. It can in rare cases cause mental confusion, seizures, or irregular heartbeat (and a doctor should be called if someone taking this drug experiences these side effects). A study has shown it doesn't actually work as a sleep aid[172], despite often being recommended as such. It may be used with older children for allergy purposes, but there are safer alternatives for many children (see home remedies section).

Cold medicine

In the fall of 2007, official sources stated that cold medicines should not be used for kids under 4[173] (some sources say under 6). They stated that these medicines do not help to banish colds any faster and may cause serious side effects, including death, in some

165   http://www.ncbi.nlm.nih.gov/pubmed/15239078
166   http://www.ncbi.nlm.nih.gov/pubmed/15239078
167   http://www.nlm.nih.gov/medlineplus/news/fullstory_131229.html
168   http://www.yalemedicalgroup.org/stw/Page.asp?PageID=STW026871
169   http://www.yalemedicalgroup.org/stw/Page.asp?PageID=STW026871
170   http://pediatrics.aappublications.org/content/119/1/e124.full
171   http://www.drugs.com/sfx/diphenhydramine-side-effects.html
172   http://www.medicineonline.com/news/10/9112/Antihistamine-Doesn-t-Help-Babies-Sleep.html
173   http://www.webmd.com/cold-and-flu/kids-cold-medicine-safety-information

children. These drugs were, in some cases, associated with unexplained infant death[174]. Cold medicines only dry up nasal secretions, they do not help the body fight off illness or get well any faster, and children do not need them.

Robitussin

Cough suppressants like this one were included in the warning on children's cold medicine back in 2007, and were also associated with the unexplained infant deaths that cold medicines were[175]. Suppressing a cough can be dangerous, because coughing is a natural response used to clear mucus out of a child's lungs. Studies also show that honey can more effectively combat coughs (and is safer) than OTC drugs[176] (although it should not be used in children under 1).

Ibuprofen

This is another drug that is commonly used to reduce fevers and pain in children. It is also known to deplete glutathione and cause liver toxicity[177]. In rare cases it is associated with chronic hepatitis[178]. It can impair normal cartilage production and also interfere with hydration[179]. There are safer ways to reduce pain.

Pepto-Bismol

This drug is in the same class as aspirin (a form of salicylate) and could induce Reye's syndrome in children, and should not be used in kids under 12[180]. It is normally used to control diarrhea, but there are safer ways to do so.

Laxatives

These drugs are questionable for anyone, as they can be habit-forming (meaning that children or adults will be unable to move their bowels without using the drugs). Side effects of common laxatives (Miralax) include gas, bloating, upset stomach, dizziness, increased sweating, rectal bleeding, and severe or bloody diarrhea[181]. A child who is experiencing constipation should seek medical help to address any potential dietary issues (food allergies or low-nutrition diets may be responsible) and laxatives should not be used without a professional's guidance.

As you can see, these drugs are not without serious side effects and in some cases, should not be used by children at all. That does not mean that children who are experiencing illness need to suffer, however. In future sections, you will see several safer home remedies to aid a child with acute illnesses. If you have any serious concerns, call a medical professional.

If you do have or wish to use any of the above medications, consult a health professional for guidance on appropriate dosing for your child's age, weight, and situation. Use the minimum recommended dosage for the shortest amount of time, and

174   http://www.medscape.com/viewarticle/586718
175   http://babygooroo.com/2008/08/study-reinforces-risks-of-cough-and-cold-medicines-in-infants-and-young-children/
176   http://www.ncbi.nlm.nih.gov/pubmed/18056558
177   http://www.ncbi.nlm.nih.gov/pmc/articles/PMC1421419/
178   http://livertox.nlm.nih.gov/Ibuprofen.htm
179   http://fellrnr.com/wiki/NSAIDs_and_Running
180   http://www.fisher-price.com/en_US/playtime/parenting/articlesandadvice/articledetail.html?article=tcm:169-18981
181   http://www.rxlist.com/miralax-drug/patient-images-side-effects.htm#sideeffects

follow up with a health professional with any questions or concerns.

The safest way to avoid OTC drug use in most cases is to have a natural health arsenal at your disposal before illness strikes, so that you are prepared for common concerns and not scrambling while your children are not feeling well. See the herbal guide for more information, and consult an alternative doctor or master herbalist with specific questions.

A NOTE ON ANTIBIOTICS AND PRESCRIPTION MEDICATION

These days, most people are aware that antibiotic resistance is a real problem and that the decision to use prescription medication is one to consider carefully. However, many parents still feel the need to *do something* when their child is sick or dealing with a problem, and many doctors want to help. Thus, medication is still overprescribed.

It's not that prescription medication of any kind should *never* be used. It's that the decision to use it must be made very carefully. Safer alternatives (dietary changes, herbal medicines, vitamin or mineral supplements) ought to be explored as initial avenues, unless a life or death situation exists. There is a time and a place for medication, but it should be after underlying issues have been examined.

Unfortunately most prescriptions are written for simple illnesses, like ear infections or sinus infections. ADHD is another common reason for children to be taking medication. In many of these cases, the medication is not needed. Antibiotics have been shown to have very little impact on ear infections, for example[182] (and may even lead to repeat infections because they wipe out good gut bacteria in the process). They've also shown to be of little benefit for sinus infections[183],[184]. Still, doctors prescribe them for these uses every day.

A fairly recent study shows that kids with ADHD are likely better helped by dietary interventions than by medication[185]. Other studies show that the youngest kids in class are more likely to be given prescriptions for it than older kids[186], suggesting that developmental maturity and not an actual illness may be responsible for the symptoms, at least in some cases.

One study shows that up to 25% of all antibiotic prescriptions are actually written for infections that are either probably or definitely viral – which antibiotics cannot help[187]. This can open up a person to more infections down the line, as well as antibiotic resistance – a serious issue, should a child ever really *need* an antibiotic. Doctors are now advising that if a diagnosis is uncertain or if a child may recover without intervention that a "wait and see" approach be taken, and that the decision to use a prescription should be made a day or two down the road, if the child isn't recovering and a more firm diagnosis can be made (i.e. that it is actually a bacterial infection).

Doctors are often not following proper prescription guidelines and are often prescribing antibiotics "just in case" or for fear of unlikely complications in order to avoid a lawsuit, some studies suggest[188]. Others may prescribe one because parents specifically ask for one, rather than taking the time (and potentially, the parent's unhappiness) to explain why an antibiotic is not needed. This is a reason to be a partner with your doctor and not ask for an antibiotic when it is unneeded as many doctors will write prescriptions to

---

182   http://www.cnn.com/2010/HEALTH/11/16/antibiotics.ear.infections/index.html
183   http://www.drugs.com/news/antibiotics-don-t-help-most-sinus-infections-study-finds-36459.html
184   http://www.sciencedaily.com/releases/2008/04/080415194352.htm
185   http://www.sciencedaily.com/releases/2008/04/080415194352.htm
186   http://bostonglobe.com/lifestyle/health-wellness/2012/11/23/youngest-kids-class-more-likely-get-adhd-drugs-study-finds/8cFhKMsjOWaxXiSVO7pliN/story.html
187   http://www.reuters.com/article/2011/11/07/us-kids-antibiotic-rxs-idUSTRE7A66U820111107
188   http://www.reuters.com/article/2011/11/07/us-kids-antibiotic-rxs-idUSTRE7A66U820111107

"CYA" so to speak.

When these drugs are overused, it is not just a concern about resistance (although this is a serious concern now, with MRSA and other resistant infections). Wiping out good gut flora on a regular basis is also associated with the development of IBD, Crohn's disease, and other bowel disorders, because of the disturbed gut flora[189]. Overuse of antibiotics, especially in young babies, may significantly increase the risk of asthma[190].

Corticosteroids, now often prescribed to relieve symptoms in addition to or instead of antibiotics (in the case of respiratory infections) are also not necessarily effective[191].

If a child is ill, first determine if it can be treated safely at home. The majority of colds, flu, sinus and ear infections, and other common childhood ailments can be. If in doubt, call the child's doctor and ask for a phone consultation with him/her or a nurse in the office. Describe the child's symptoms, ask for ways to treat at home and what to look for as far as "when it's serious." Do not make an appointment unless the medical professional feels that it is actually warranted in that child's case.

If an appointment is necessary, ask for diagnostic tests to figure out what ailment the child actually has and if antibiotics are really indicated before accepting a prescription. Discuss other treatment options if possible. Studies show that good communication and blood tests can reduce the over prescription problem[192]. Although blood tests are not fun for the child or parent, they can more accurately determine if a drug is needed – and given the serious issue with overuse, are warranted if a child is suspected of having something serious enough to require a drug.

In the case of "chronic" conditions like IBD or ADHD, look into dietary intervention and other alternative therapies before accepting a prescription. These conditions can often be managed with diet changes, probiotics, and other non-drug therapy. Be wary of any doctor who immediately prescribes a drug or who suggests that a drug is the only solution.

In general, any doctor who suggests (especially in a chronic or minor acute situation – *not* a life-threatening or serious situation) that a drug is the *only* option should not be taken seriously. Seek a second opinion. Again – this is not talking about a truly serious situation, in which case the drug may be the best or only option. The doctor should be willing to explain to you why the drug is needed in a way that you can understand.

If your child is prescribed a drug, and you believe it to be necessary, make sure to ask questions. Is the child being given a low dose to start? What side effects should you be looking for? Is this the safest drug for this particular condition, given your child's history? Is there a package insert that you can read? Make sure your questions are answered thoroughly.

Read through the package insert you are given and know exactly how the drug should be taken and what side effects (both minor and serious) to look for. If you see any side effects, especially serious ones or potential allergic reactions, call the doctor or pharmacist immediately.

189   http://specialty.pharmacytimes.com/clinical/Crohnsdisease/-Overprescription-of-Antibiotics-
       Increases-Risk-of-IBD-
190   http://www.sciencedaily.com/releases/2011/01/110127090152.htm
191   http://www.sciencedaily.com/releases/2012/08/120807132205.htm
192   http://www.sciencedaily.com/releases/2009/05/090521112706.htm

Be sure to take the drug exactly as prescribed. One of the reasons for antibiotic-resistant infections is because the antibiotics are not taken as prescribed – they are taken for only a few days, and then stopped when the patient is feeling better. Or, doses are skipped, doubled, or otherwise taken improperly. Do not misuse a medication, and do not ever share a drug with someone else. It is illegal to share a prescription drug with someone for whom it was not prescribed – not to mention potentially dangerous. Drugs are serious and should be treated this way when they are needed.

Always follow up with a health professional as requested, especially if you see side effects or the symptoms have not abated by the time the drug course is finished. Consider probiotic use in between doses of antibiotics (not with them, but several hours after/before a dose) to combat the issue of potential yeast infections.

The decision to use drugs is one that should not be taken lightly, but which should be made through a careful examination by a qualified health professional with any necessary tests run. If the child is found to have a serious problem, then drug therapy should be considered. Continue reading to learn how to treat self-limiting conditions at home (always remembering that if in doubt, call a doctor to ask questions).

BOOSTING THE IMMUNE SYSTEM NATURALLY

If you're sufficiently worried about how to keep your kids healthy after reading the last two sections, don't be afraid (or overwhelmed). There are many natural ways to boost a child's immune system so that they get sick less often and over all are healthier. It's not 'use mainstream medicine' or be miserable!

Breastfeeding as a newborn, and into toddlerhood, is one of the most important factors. Breastmilk functions as an immune system for a newborn who doesn't yet have one; in fact, breast milk contains most of the factors that the newborn is missing[193]. It is protective against a number of respiratory and intestinal illnesses[194] and helps to develop the newborn's immature gut[195], playing a strong role in the ultimate development of the newborn's immune system.

Breast milk continues to be an important part of a child's diet even beyond the first year. It especially can provide needed fats and vitamin A to developing bodies[196] and some sources show that immunological benefits become more concentrated, and that extended breastfeeding is protective against childhood cancers, diabetes, obesity, strep throat, and several other common illnesses[197]. Breastfeeding until a child self-weans is ideal, which may be anywhere between 2 and 7 years.

For children who aren't breastfeeding or who are past breastfeeding age, there are additional ways to boost the immune system.

Vitamin D is an important part of the immune system. Vitamin D receptors are present on important immune cells and can help them respond to threats in the body[198]...or not, if the person is deficient[199]. Cod liver oil is one of the best sources of vitamin D[200] because it is food-based and well absorbed by the body. Of course, the very best source of vitamin D is sun exposure, which must occur without any sunscreen to be effective. The best sun exposure to produce vitamin D, yet minimize one's risk of sun-associated cancers and other illnesses is right around noon, when the UVB rays (which produce vitamin D) are the strongest[201].

Vitamin A is another important factor in a strong immune system. The ratio of vitamin A to vitamin D is the blood is critical (too much vitamin D alone can lead to high calcium levels and kidney stones) and can boost the immune system safely[202]. Adequate vitamin A has also been associated with decreased morbidity (the chances of getting sick) and mortality (the chances of dying) in a number of different studies[203].

---

193   http://www.fmhs.uaeu.ac.ae/neonatal/iss003/p2.pdf
194   http://www.fmhs.uaeu.ac.ae/neonatal/iss003/p2.pdf
195   http://www.medicinabiointegrata.com/doc/probiotici/Microflora%20intestinale%20nel%20bambino.pdf
196   http://kellymom.com/ages/older-infant/ebf-benefits/
197   http://www.whale.to/a/steinkraus.html
198   http://www.ncbi.nlm.nih.gov/pubmed/21527855
199   http://www.jabfm.org/content/22/6/698.full
200   http://www.ncbi.nlm.nih.gov/pubmed/12897318
201   http://www.ncbi.nlm.nih.gov/pubmed/18348449
202   http://www.westonaprice.org/blogs/cmasterjohn/2012/01/22/new-evidence-of-synergy-between-vitamins-a-and-d-protection-against-autoimmune-diseases/
203   http://www.bmj.com/content/343/bmj.d5094

Vitamin C may play an important role as well (although it is important to avoid synthetic sources). Vitamin C seems to boost an important component of the immune system, IgA, which helps to prevent viral infections[204]. It would not hurt to consume extra vitamin C-rich foods during the winter months.

Probiotics also play an important role in the immune system. Gut flora affects strongly whether a person can handle infection well, without getting sick – or at least, without getting very sick. Strains from lactobacilli and bifidobacterium are especially effective at boosting the immune system and reducing the risk of several different illnesses and conditions (both chronic and acute)[205]. Probiotics can even interact with the body and prime the immune system and mobilize important defenses to prevent disease[206]. Taking a high-quality probiotic supplement that contains several different strains or consuming a wide variety of probiotic foods can improve the immune system.

Moderate exercise is also beneficial. Children should be encouraged to be physical and to move around every day for a period of time. Exercise increases the body's ability to naturally "detox" as well as moving important white blood cells through the body faster, allowing them to recognize and kill infections faster[207]. Plus, exercise in many other ways to promote health.

In general, avoiding nutrient deficiencies through an excellent diet and supplementing with fermented cod liver oil (which has the proper ratio of vitamin A to vitamin D in naturally-occurring, not synthetic form) will help to keep the body healthy. See the sections on food and nutrition for more about a healthy diet for children.

More ways of boosting the immune system under certain circumstances (i.e. during illness) will be discussed in later sections of the book.

204   http://profiles.nlm.nih.gov/ps/access/MMBBRN.pdf
205   http://www.ncbi.nlm.nih.gov/pubmed/19442167
206   http://www.ncbi.nlm.nih.gov/pmc/articles/PMC3023613/
207   http://www.nlm.nih.gov/medlineplus/ency/article/007165.htm

SUPPLEMENTS

Should your child receive supplements? If so, which kind? If not...why not?

Most doctors these days recommend a basic multivitamin as well as a vitamin D supplement, usually drops. These may not be your child's best option, however. Some studies show that synthetic vitamins are not as well absorbed as natural forms. Plus, naturally occurring vitamins occur in groups, and not in isolation[208]. Since vitamins may compete for receptors in the body, megadoses of one may lead to deficiencies in another[209].

Still, there's a lot of evidence that adequate vitamins and minerals can help to ward off any number of diseases, not to mention helping children grow and develop properly. What's a parent to do?

There are a few safe, non-synthetic supplements that may be beneficial to children.

Fermented Cod Liver Oil

This supplement is one of my favorites and one that I make sure that I have around all the time. It is a good source of vitamin A, vitamin D, omega-3 fatty acids (like DHA and EPA), and many other enzymes and nutrients. Omega-3s have been shown to be beneficial to children's brain development[210],[211]. It has long been used to protect children's health and reduce the incidence of disease[212]. Some studies show that up to 4000 IU per day of vitamin D is needed[213]. As mentioned earlier in the book, vitamin D is safest when taken in conjunction with vitamin A, and both naturally occur in cod liver oil.

This has been our experience over the last few years and it's something I'd recommend to every family. In some cases it has been able to stop a cold in its tracks by taking extra at the first sign of symptoms, and as in the study cited previously (121) we experienced fewer respiratory illnesses when we took it regularly.

Probiotics

Friendly bacteria is incredibly important to our gut health, and our gut health affects our immune system[214]. These days, we don't get enough from food in most cases (which is ideal). The most common source of probiotics for most kids is yogurt (however, the yogurt most children eat, which is commercial contains sweeteners, flavors, and colors, does not have enough live, active cultures to be very beneficial). For some children, probiotic supplements are the best option, especially if they do not like or the family chooses not to consume probiotic foods (like kombucha, milk and water kefir, and fermented fruits and vegetables).

A good probiotic is raw and food-based. It should contain 5 – 10 billion live cultures

---

208   http://www.nlm.nih.gov/medlineplus/ency/article/007165.htm
209   http://journals.cambridge.org/download.php?file=%2F13617_324721309E50DD8691A6EEA70C9
       EE260_journals__NRR_NRR13_02_S0954422400000706a.pdf&cover=Y&code=09ca5df6bf33b2b3
       1d84a553e6b92ef1
210   http://www.ox.ac.uk/media/news_stories/2012/120709_1.html
211   http://www.sciencedaily.com/releases/2008/07/080709161922.htm
212   http://www.jacn.org/content/29/6/559.abstract
213   http://ucsdnews.ucsd.edu/pressrelease/vitamin_d_deficiency_linked_to_type_1_diabetes
214   http://www.pnas.org/content/107/1/454.full

and have several different probiotic strains[215], especially s. boulardii, b. infantis, and l. acidophilus. Other strains in the lactobacillus family are also good. Read labels carefully before selecting a product, and choose one that is refrigerated; products can vary widely in composition and price. We have chosen Garden of Life probiotic supplements when we use a supplement at all.

What about fish oil?

Some parents like to offer their children fish oil because it is more readily available, less expensive, and because it has been shown to contain beneficial omega-3 fatty acids. This is not ideal, however. Fish oil does have these benefits, but it does not contain any vitamin D. Cod liver oil, on the other hand, contains the same omega-3s and also contains vitamin D[216]. Many fish oils on the market are also purified and have synthetic vitamins added to them. A traditionally fermented cod liver oil is going to provide a much greater benefit than a standard fish oil.

What about vitamin D drops?

Many parents are told they must supplement their babies and young children with vitamin D drops. These are certainly convenient, as most brands require only a single drop to get 400 IU per day, which is the "recommended" dose by most pediatricians. New research shows this amount may not be adequate. However, these drops are usually derived from lanolin and are essentially a highly processed[217], synthetic form of D3. The lanolin is extracted from the wool and exposed to ultraviolet light to create the vitamin D3 in a lab[218], which is then extracted and purified (often using chemicals) before being mixed with some type of oil. This oil may be coconut, palm, soy, or another "carrier" oil. Lanolin is used because it is cheap and easily available. It is not a whole foods source of vitamin D and not ideal.

There are no studies on this type of vitamin D showing that it is absorbed properly – there have been assumptions made because it is "oil based" and therefore must be similar to cod liver oil. All studies I located about the effectiveness of vitamin D used cod liver oil. Better is to supplement the breastfeeding mother or to rub cod liver oil on baby's bottom until s/he is old enough to take it orally (8 months or so, whenever solids are started).

A note on RDA

It is important to remember when assessing supplement labels, if you are looking at any commercial brands, that the RDA listed on the label is *not* the recommended optimal amount. The RDA, or "Recommended Daily Allowance" is the minimum amount required to stave off deficiency and any related illnesses. Most children (and adults) could benefit from amounts several times what are listed on the label. However, this needs to come largely in food form, not supplement form, so that the person does not inadvertently cause deficiencies in one area by taking megadoses in others, as stated above. *Most nutrients should come from foods; supplements should be used to "top off" where needed.*

I do not give or recommend any other supplements on a regular basis. I do occasionally

215   http://www.aafp.org/afp/2008/1101/p1073.html
216   http://www.jabfm.org/content/18/5/445.1.full
217   http://en.wikipedia.org/wiki/Cholecalciferol
218   http://en.wikipedia.org/wiki/Cholecalciferol

choose to use a liquid herbal multivitamin[219] and topical magnesium chloride, but these are offered to children typically only if they are ill or have been exposed to illness. Adults benefit more from these in my opinion, although there is no harm in using them with children in small amounts. Ask a health professional for specific advice for your family.

If your children have specific deficiencies or nutritional needs due to any special health conditions, please seek the advice of a health professional before choosing any supplements. Your children may not do well with the above options, or may need additional supplements to meet their needs. If your child does have a medical condition, do not add to or change his/her supplements without consulting your child's doctor, as certain medical conditions result in chronic deficiencies or levels which are too high, and supplementing could be potentially dangerous.

Healthy children without medical conditions should do well with the above options in most cases, but ask a health professional if in doubt.

---

219   http://www.modernalternativemama.com/blog/2012/01/23/monday-health-wellness-herbal-multivitamin-tincture/

FEVERS

· ·

Fevers are very common in childhood, yet few symptoms make parents worry more. Parents have been taught to fear fevers, to see them as bad, and to try to lower them as quickly as possible. Unfortunately, most parents don't know why fevers occur, what is *really* a "high fever" and how (and why) to work *with* fevers instead of against them to help their children recover.

These days, parents consider 101 – 102 to be a "high fever" and will medicate. Most doctors will recommend medicating fevers at this level, as well. But is it necessary?

A fever's function in the body is to kill the infection by making the body inhospitable to the infectious agent[220]. If the fever is artificially lowered, then the fever cannot do its job to kill whatever is making the child sick. Fevers become somewhat worrisome around 104, and potentially dangerous around 105 to 106[221]. Fevers much higher than this can cause brain damage, but they are incredibly rare and are usually brought on by medication, sunstroke, or some outside cause (not natural infection). This is quite a bit higher than what most parents consider "high!"

Many parents are scared of febrile seizures occurring during fever. They are not always due to high fevers and do not typically cause any brain damage or other permanent damage. Most of the time, febrile seizures occur because of how quickly a fever rises rather than how high it is, and using medication to try to force the fever down can make febrile seizures more likely as the body fights to spike the fever higher and faster, especially as the medication is wearing off. Children who have multiple seizures, seizures that affect only one part of the body, or which last longer than 15 minutes should be seen[222]. Otherwise a quick call to the doctor to rule out the need for a visit is probably sufficient. Febrile seizures are far scarier for parents than for the child.

It is also true that fevers of unknown cause are often due to viral illness[223], which is not responsive to antibiotics anyway (i.e. no need to rush to the doctor for medication to treat). Prolonged high fevers might be due to bacterial infection and children who are miserable in other ways – dehydrated, unable to keep down fluids, etc. – should see a doctor, but for fever alone it is not necessary.

To treat a fever, in general, do nothing. Taking a child's temperature is not even necessary if the child is over 6 months old (young babies with immature immune systems who are suspected of having fevers should be checked and a call to the doctor should be made, as it is much more dangerous for them than older ones). A child who feels hot and dry usually is feverish; a child who is hot and sweaty is simply hot. (Sweat is the body's way of cooling the body; a feverish child's body will not be attempting to cool off.)

More important than the fever are the accompanying symptoms and the behavior of the child. Even if the fever is high, if the child seems "okay" – is playing, drinking, possibly eating a bit, resting quietly – leave him/her alone. If the child is miserable, screaming, inconsolable, lethargic, unable to keep down fluids, dehydrated, etc. then a call to a doctor may be warranted, but it is because of the additional symptoms, *not* the fever

---

220   http://www.scientificamerican.com/article.cfm?id=what-causes-a-fever
221   http://www.mindspring.com/~drwarren/fever.htm
222   http://www.ncbi.nlm.nih.gov/pubmedhealth/PMH0001975/
223   http://www.medscape.com/viewarticle/773888

itself.

Provide a feverish child with comfort – a warm bath (cool will make the body work harder to maintain the fever and may make it worse), snuggling, nursing (if an infant/toddler), extra rest, fluids, and so on. A bit of lavender or peppermint essential oil may help to alleviate discomfort and facilitate rest. Additional comfort methods may be used depending on additional symptoms present. Call a doctor if the fever is very high, prolonged, or accompanied by worrying symptoms.

(Be aware that a common infection called roseola can produce high fevers of 104 – 105 that last several days, but the child will be acting "well," eating and playing mostly normally. This is viral and also not a concern. Most parents do not know it is roseola until the characteristic rash erupts after the fever breaks. Many young children do get this at one point or another.)

If other comfort methods are needed, there are some suggestions below. If a child can rest and is not miserable due to the high temperature (young children have higher fevers than do adults and also tolerate them better, so what would be difficult for a parent is not necessarily difficult for the child – watch his/her reaction), leave the child alone. If, however, the child is miserable and unable to rest due to the fever, try some of these just to help the child sleep.

Other Comfort Methods:

- **Calcium** – It has been suggested (both by an alternative doctor to me personally and via internet research) that calcium deficiencies can lead to fevers, and that giving calcium lactate in pill form every 30 minutes until the fever breaks can be helpful. Depending on the cause this may or may not be the best idea.

- **Peppermint essential oil** – Mixed with a carrier oil and placed on the feet to help relieve fever.

- **Lemon socks** – Some suggest that the properties of lemon can reduce discomfort without reducing a fever prematurely[224].

- **Warm bath** -- Place the child in a comfortably warm bath. A few drops of lavender essential oil for relaxation can be used. Get in the tub with a young child (under 18 months or so; snuggling with you will relax him/her too). A cool bath should not be used because it will cause the child to shiver in an attempt to keep the fever high and may even spike it higher.

- **Epsom salts** – These can be added to a warm bath to relax and also detox the child, helping to fight the infection faster.

- **Chiropractic** – In some cases, an adjustment can help the body to function more efficiently and end the fever faster (because it isn't needed, not artificially soon).

In general, let a feverish child rest and talk to a medical professional if the child's symptoms or demeanor are worrying. Do not worry about a fever alone in a child who is resting and drinking well.

---

224   http://www.holisticsquid.com/lemon-socks-for-a-fever/

COLDS AND FLU

What kid doesn't get a cold from time to time? Or even the flu? Even healthy children may expect 1 – 2 colds per year and this is not a sign of a problem. (Catching "every cold that goes around" is different and not good!)

No parent wants to see their child suffer, so many want to "do something" to help their child – offer cold or cough medication, sore throat remedies, even antibiotics. Please check back in the sections on OTC and prescription drugs to see why these are not a good idea, especially for young children.

The majority of colds and flu can be handled at home. Even if a child is ill enough to require a doctor's care, they can generally only offer supportive care. Of course, if a child is actually struggling to breathe, is breathing very rapidly, is very young, or has any sign of complications (high fever, unable to keep food/liquid down, etc.) then a doctor should be consulted. Fortunately these complications are rare.

For run-of-the-mill colds and flu, the following remedies may offer some relief:

- **Elderberry** – Certain compounds in elderberry may cut the duration of colds and flu in half as well as relieving some symptoms[225]. Elderberry syrup should be given at the first sign of a cold or flu and given a few times a day until symptoms ease – about 1 tsp. for children and 1 tbsp. for adults (although, as a food, an overdose is highly unlikely). Try making your own[226] (swap honey for cane sugar for babies under a year).

- **Ginger** – This remedy is safe for all ages. Make some hot tea from fresh ginger and serve with honey and lemon juice (if desired). This can help sore throats, coughs, and sinus pressure.

- **Rosemary or eucalyptus essential oils** – These oils can help open breathing passages and improve breathing. They can be put in diffusers, humidifiers, in a bowl of steaming water (place a towel over the older child's head as they lean over the bowl and breathe in the vapors), or a drop on the front of the child's clothes. They can also be mixed with coconut oil and spread on the feet for a homemade "vapor rub."

- **Breastmilk** – Especially for younger babies, this is the safest and most effective remedy. Squirt breastmilk up their noses, which will help to clear up the congestion (breastmilk actually breaks it down). Then, use a nasal aspirator to suck out whatever loose congestion there is so they can breathe better. If milk is expressed, it can be squirted up any child's nose with a syringe.

- **Saline solution** – If breastmilk is not available, use a saline solution to try to break up congestion instead. A small amount of baking soda (about ¼ tsp.) in a cup of water can be used, or there are commercial sprays available.

- **Neti pot** – This is for older children, age 5 or so and up. Use only filtered water in

---

225   http://israel21c.org/health/study-shows-israeli-elderberry-extract-effective-against-avian-flu/
226   http://www.modernalternativemama.com/blog/2013/01/21/monday-health-and-wellness-ulti-
       mate-elderberry-syrup/

these, as tap water may be contaminated with amoebas and there have been scattered reports of serious infections from using neti pots with tap water. Mix in a little baking soda and use the neti pot to clear the sinuses.

- **Capsaicin** – Using some form of capsaicin (found in peppers) can open breathing passages and drain the sinuses. Think spicy foods. Horseradish is also effective in a similar way.
- **Garlic** – Garlic is naturally antibacterial. The best way to take it is a fresh, crushed clove on a spoon, covered with honey. This is often too strong for children; it can also be mixed with coconut oil and spread on the feet instead.
- **Honey** – Children over a year can simply swallow a spoonful of honey to help quiet coughs, especially at night.
- **Homemade cough/cold syrup**[227] – We found this was fairly effective at reducing cold symptoms if taken at the onset of symptoms. The herbs fenugreek and slippery elm work together to both increase mucus production and also clear mucus from the body faster, thus helping to clear the infection itself faster. It can be given without honey or subbing cane sugar for babies 6 – 12 months.
- **Epsom salt baths** – This can boost the body's magnesium levels and also help detox, resulting in the child feeling a bit better, resting easier, and hopefully feeling better sooner.
- **FCLO** – Fermented cod liver oil boosts the body's vitamin A and D levels, which can help the body to fight off infection.
- **Arnica** – Sometimes body aches are part of a cold or flu. Arnica is a homeopathic remedy for muscle pain, which may ease this symptom. It can be used in pellet form or as a rub.

Most of these remedies can safely be used for any age, and certainly for children over age 1. Breastmilk is the safest remedy for the smallest ones, along with plenty of nursing and snuggles. Most remedies can easily be used in combination as well. Choose what works best for your family; some notice more help from one than another. Over time you will create an "arsenal" of remedies that work best for you.

Our preference is for the essential oils in a humidifier, breastmilk up the nose, ginger tea, and FCLO. Sometimes we use the cough/cold syrup. We rarely use the other remedies personally, but everyone is different.

---

227   http://www.modernalternativemama.com/blog/2011/10/24/monday-health-wellness-home-made-cough-and-cold-syrup.html

STOMACH VIRUSES

Our family unfortunately experienced this in December, 2012, right around the time I was writing this book. One of the major ways to help someone experiencing a stomach virus is to rehydrate them properly. That is, to replenish electrolytes and not just fluids. Store-bought options are not very good for this as many contain artificial colors, flavors, and sweeteners that can exacerbate nausea rather than improve it. Luckily there are homemade options that are safer and beneficial. I cannot describe the relief I personally felt from drinking such a concoction when I was sick – it was almost immediate and it helped so much.

The aftermath of caring for someone with a stomach virus is just as important as caring for them while it is happening. When someone experiences ongoing vomiting and/or diarrhea, they do become somewhat dehydrated and their healthy gut flora is washed out of the body. It is important to help restore and replenish this over the next several days.

At the first signs of a stomach virus, allow the body to do what it needs to do – purge. This is not fun for anyone, but sometimes the body needs to rid itself of something. Suppressing it is probably not the way to go. There are ways to attempt to prevent vomiting (which I will cover below), but in my experience this actually prolonged the illness rather than solving the problem. It depends on the person and the cause but be aware that sometimes, it is just better to allow the symptoms.

Once the vomiting has slowed or stopped (no vomiting for at least one hour), small sips of liquid can be offered. After a couple of hours of liquid being tolerated, small bits of food can be offered, if the person wants to eat. If they don't want to eat, don't push it on them. Don't push liquids too quickly because an unsettled stomach will result in further vomiting, which increases the risk of dehydration. It is better to offer nothing than risk more vomiting.

A person who is experiencing severe vomiting (vomiting occurring every few minutes after there is nothing left but stomach acid; for whom nausea cannot stop; which lasts for several hours without slowing) or who is dehydrated or otherwise experiencing complications may be better off seeking medical attention so they can get an IV for rehydration and/or anti-nausea drugs. In most cases this is not necessary but for some it will be.

Here are some remedies that may help:

- **Bentonite Clay** – Taken as a capsule or mixed into a drink, it binds with any toxins or "yuck" in the system and helps to carry it out.
- **Activated Charcoal** – Works similarly to bentonite clay and is usually available locally. Good for food poisoning.
- **Ginger** – Has anti-nausea properties and is safe for all ages. Take in tea or pill form.
- **Peppermint** – The essential oil used for smelling (dabbed on the hand, diluted; in a diffuser, etc.) can help relieve nausea.
- **Rehydration drink** – 3 c. water, juice of ½ lemon, 2 tbsp. honey, ¼ tsp. sea salt

mixed together. If desired, boil the water with 3 – 4 slices ginger before proceeding with the recipe for a ginger-lemon flavor. This helps reduce nausea and replenish needed electrolytes.

- **Garlic** – Garlic mixed with coconut oil (freshly crushed) and spread on the feet can help kill any bacteria or other junk in the system, helping the person to get well faster.

- **Lemon balm** – This herb has some anti-nausea properties. It is naturally caffeine-free, so tea can be made and offered to someone of any age.

- **Bone broth** – Homemade, real bone broth can help to soothe an irritated digestive tract, as well as pulling out some of the "yuck" in the system and providing much-needed nutrients.

- **Epsom salt bath** – A hot bath with Epsom salts can also help to pull the junk out of the system through the skin and help the person to feel better. Alternately, use bentonite clay for a bath, but it's quite messy.

- **Nux Vomica** – This is a homeopathic remedy known to stop vomiting in some cases (check with a trained homeopath to see if this is the right remedy for you).

- **Ipecac (homeopathic)** – While syrup of ipecac induces vomiting, the homeopathic variety has been shown to slow or stop vomiting (check with a trained homeopath to see if this is the right remedy for you).

- **Starch** – Starchy foods like potatoes or even products made with white flour may help to absorb digestive juices and settle the stomach. Choose varieties without additional unhealthy ingredients. (We chose Snack Factory Pretzel Crisps mostly recently.) Use very temporarily.

- **Probiotics** – After a stomach virus, especially one that includes a lot of diarrhea, the gut flora is "cleared out" of your system. Some research shows the appendix's job is to help repopulate the gut, but you can help by consuming additional probiotics. Yogurt, kombucha, kefir, fermented fruits/veggies, or probiotic supplements are good. Don't push these too quickly especially milk-based varieties, but include them once the stomach is settled and the person wants to begin eating again.

Try a variety of the above remedies, especially once the vomiting slows. Allow recovery to happen slowly, and once the person is feeling better, drink quite a bit of fluid, especially the rehydration drink. The body needs to regain both the good gut flora and the proper electrolyte balance, and may have additional "detoxing" to do. (It's pretty stressful on the body to vomit and otherwise "purge" so much.) Continue to rest for the next few days until all signs are back to normal. Watch urine to see if it is darker yellow than usual and if so, increase fluids (even after the person is feeling better).

Luckily, stomach viruses don't happen too often and if handled properly, can be a good way for the body to purge the "junk" and resettle itself.

EAR INFECTIONS

Ear infections are one of the most common reasons for parents to visit a doctor each year. They're very uncomfortable and children who have them often don't rest well and cry a lot. Parents want to make their children feel better (understandably).

The most common "treatment" is antibiotics. Unfortunately, many ear infections are viral and antibiotics cannot help them. Even for ear infections that are bacterial, they often clear up in the same number of days with or without antibiotics. Using antibiotics may also lead to recurrent ear infections or other, more serious infections because they wipe out the good gut flora in addition to the ear infection bacteria. If possible, skip the antibiotics and try some of the remedies below.

- **Garlic oil** – Mix a freshly crushed clove of garlic with olive oil and allow it to sit for about five minutes. Strain the oil to remove any trace of garlic chunks. Put 3 – 5 drops in the affected ear (while the child is laying on his/her side) and gently tug on the earlobe to get the oil in. Allow this to sit for about five minutes, then help the child turn over so the ear can drain.

- **Mullein** – Use this herb infused in oil and dropped into the child's ear, as described above. It may be combined with the garlic to be especially effective.

- **Onion** – Cut an onion and place the cut side against the ear (a large piece, so it can't go inside). Use a piece of gauze to hold it in place. Change it every several hours. The onion juices will help draw out the infection.

- **Eucalyptus oil** – Mix eucalyptus essential oil with a carrier oil and place a few drops in the ear. Follow the same procedure as with the garlic oil, allowing it to sit and then drain.

- **Chiropractic** – An adjustment may change the angle of the tubes in the ears, allowing them to drain properly and clearing the infection. (An infection happens in the first place because the tubes get blocked, the fluid can't drain, and it becomes infected. This causes the pain and full feeling associated with ear infections.)

- **Colloidal silver** – A few drops of silver in the ears, as with the garlic oil, may help to clear the infection.

- **Hydrogen peroxide** – A few drops of hydrogen peroxide in the ears may help to dry up any fluid that is present. This is especially helpful in a case like swimmer's ear.

- **FCLO** – Boost the child's overall immune system with extra fermented cod liver oil for vitamins A and D.

Try combining a few of the above remedies – not at the exact same time, but at different times throughout the day. An alternative doctor's herbal suggestions may also be beneficial. There are many different herbal anti-bacterial supplements that can be used orally or topically to help clear ear infections if the child is struggling.

Essential oils in a diffuser in the child's room may also be beneficial.

CUTS AND SCRAPES

Kids play...and kids fall down. Most of these falls are minor and lead to small cuts and scrapes, but nothing serious. Obviously, a child who has a serious wound – a broken bone, a cut that is bleeding heavily, etc. – should be seen by a doctor. But for your average skinned knee, there are several home remedies that are safe and beneficial.

A typical antibiotic ointment is not necessary in most cases and may be detrimental. Skip the over-the-counter creams in favor of the ideas below.

- **Soap and water** – Nothing beats plain soap and water for cleaning out a cut. Try using a castile soap that is based on healthy oils and contains no additional ingredients. Rinse and gently wash the cut to keep it clean and remove any bacteria.

- **Cotton gauze** – Keep cotton gauze pads around to wrap a bleeding injury and tape them in place to keep the cut clean and dry, especially if it is larger or deeper. Gauze can also be used to stop bleeding or keep bleeding to a minimum on more serious injuries.

- **Comfrey** – This is an herb that helps to soothe and heal skin. Use a salve based on comfrey or make a strong tea from comfrey and pour it on a cloth (cooled) and use it as a compress.

- **Calendula** – This is another soothing herb. Use it as a salve to help the skin.

- **Tea tree oil** – Dilute to 2% in a carrier oil and put a few drops on the cut to kill any bacteria. This may be too strong for some.

- **Lavender oil** – Dilute to 2% in a carrier oil and use to kill bacteria or to help soothe and heal the skin. This is especially valuable for burns.

- **Arnica** – As a salve it can reduce pain, bruising and swelling. Used homeopathically (orally) it can do the same. Try using it both ways for more serious cuts or scrapes.

- **Ice** – Plain old ice (wrapped in a towel) can help to reduce swelling and pain associated with injury.

- **Epsom salts** – A soak in Epsom salts in warm water can reduce swelling and pain associated with injury. Use a foot bath or a tub bath, depending on affected area and size of injury.

- **Hypericum** – This is a homeopathic remedy that may reduce swelling, bruising, and pain.

- **Honey** – Honey covering a wound can help draw out bacteria and promote healing faster. Studies have shown that honey is superior to keeping infection at bay compared to antibiotic creams. Best is raw honey.

There are many ways to help small injuries. Use as many of the above as needed. Keeping the cut clean while healing is the most important.

SKIN RASHES

Children can experience a lot of funny-looking rashes on their skin as they're growing. Many of these are harmless; some are not. Some are more common than others. How can parents decide what's a problem and what isn't – and what to do about it?

It is impossible to cover all the possibilities for skin rashes here, so if you have a concern about a rash your child has, ask a medical professional for help in diagnosing it. Once you have identified it positively, you may choose to look for an alternative remedy – or you may decide to go with another course of treatment.

Poison Ivy

In the summer time, children who play outside may be exposed to poison ivy. It's a red, incredibly itchy rash that may blister. The best treatment method is prevention – either by staying away from known areas of poison ivy, or by taking a *cool* bath or shower and using castile soap immediately after exposure. Never take a warm or hot shower, because this will open the pores and allow the poison to penetrate the skin, increasing the severity of the rash. There are several additional remedies if the child gets a rash anyway:

- **Oatmeal baths** – Oatmeal in a bath can help to soothe the skin rash and calm the inflammation and make the itching better.
- **Jewelweed** – This is a plant that's often found growing near poison ivy. It should be picked fresh and crushed, and the leaves should be rubbed onto the poison ivy. This remedy usually works very well.
- **Plantain** – This is a plant that grows almost everywhere as it's a common "weed." The leaves are wide and flat (this is different from the banana-like "plantains" found in a grocery store). The crushed leaves can be put on the skin and used to soothe the poison ivy as well.
- **Bentonite Clay** – A paste made from clay can be put on the rash and it can absorb some of the poison and help to soothe the rash.
- **Bryonia** – This is a homeopathic remedy that is known to help in some poison ivy cases.
- **FCLO** – Fermented cod liver oil contains high levels of vitamin A and D, which can calm inflammation in the body, including a reaction to poison ivy. We have personally used this with success as part of treatment.
- **Ginger** – This herb, prepared as a tea (fresh is ideal) also is known to combat inflammation in the body and may help calm the poison ivy reaction.

Eczema

This is an incredibly common cause of skin rashes in children. It's a flat, red, itchy rash that is kind of non-specific (no 'spots' or blotches) and it often appears on the arms, legs, or torso and may be in multiple locations. Unfortunately, most doctors consider eczema to be "normal" and not a cause for concern. However, eczema is usually associated with some type of allergy – food allergy, environmental allergy, etc. It is possible, and ideal, to get rid of eczema entirely by addressing the root cause.

My daughter had terrible eczema as a baby. It was all over her hands, legs, and torso and she'd wake up screaming and scratching. Once we addressed the food issues causing it, it went away – and never returned. See the sections on allergies for more information on addressing eczema by helping allergies.

In the mean time, there are some ways to help the child feel better.

- **Avocado oil** – Rub avocado oil into the skin to relieve the itching. Jojoba oil can also be used. Skip coconut oil, because it can be drying.
- **Oatmeal baths** – Add oatmeal to a bath to nourish the child's skin.
- **Shea butter** – Try a shea-butter based lotion (with no chemical additives; plant extracts and other plant-based oils are okay) after a bath.
- **Ginger** – Try as a tea; it's anti-inflammatory and may help calm the rash.
- **Skip baths** – Bathe less often, so that the skin has a chance to produce natural oils that aren't washed away.
- **Natural body wash** – When you do bathe your child, use only a natural body wash, not something commercial that contains detergents and other harsh ingredients (even baby washes often do). See in the Environment section about personal care products that are safe.

Ring Worm

This is a somewhat common fungal infection, which is usually diagnosed by its characteristic red, ring-shaped appearance as a skin rash. It is usually treated with OTC anti-fungal creams, but can be treated with several home remedies as well.

- **Tea tree oil** – This is a powerful anti-fungal essential oil. It should be mixed with coconut oil to about a 2% dilution and spread on the affected area.
- **Coconut oil** – Besides being spread on the rash (which can soften it and lessen itching), it can also be taken internally to fight the fungal infection.
- **Turmeric** – This root has a lot of beneficial properties (some say it is even anti-cancer). The juice from the fresh root can be rubbed onto the rash itself, or it can be mixed with honey and taken internally to combat the fungal infection.
- **Bentonite clay** – Made into a paste and spread over the rash, this may be beneficial in combating the rash.
- **Mustard seed** – Crush mustard seeds and mix with filtered water to make a paste; spread on the rash to help get rid of it.

Roseola

This is a common childhood ailment that can sometimes alarm parents – but it is harmless. It starts out usually with a high fever (103 – 105), yet the child is usually playing and eating and acting mostly normal. This often mystifies parents. Some children have high enough fevers that they become tired and lay around a bit more, and may not have much appetite, but they usually do not seem very sick. The fever lasts 4 – 5 days, and after it breaks, a characteristic red, blotchy rash spreads over the skin. By this time the child is feeling and acting back to normal, typically. Many children get this before age 5. Once the rash begins, there is nothing else to do but wait – it is not itchy and the child usually feels normal again. The rash may last hours to a few days.

The treatment for this is supportive in nature.

- **Fluids** – The child may not feel like eating much, so offer fluids. Try plain water, caffeine-free herbal teas, or the electrolyte drink recipe mentioned in the Stomach Viruses section. If the child is still nursing, offer this.
- **Warm baths** – If the fever is making the child very uncomfortable, try a warm bath. Do not us a *cool* bath, as this will fight against the fever and cause the body to spike the temperature higher. It also makes a febrile seizure more likely. The goal is to help the child relax, not bring down the fever.
- **Light meals** – If the child does want to eat, offer whatever the child seems to want. Otherwise, fresh fruit or freshly-squeezed juices or a few whole grain, soaked crackers may be a good idea. A body that is healing needs to focus on that, not digestion.
- **Rest** – Allow the child to rest and sleep as needed.

Yeast

Having yeast can cause a rash as well – usually in the diaper area, but also in other areas at times (usually creases, folds of skin like around the top of the legs, backs of knees, elbows). The yeast rash is usually bright red and itchy. It can also appear in the mouth as white patches, which is then called thrush. If a baby has a yeast rash – common after a round of antibiotics in baby or nursing mom – it will usually show up in multiple locations eventually (bottom and mouth). It can be hard to cure in some cases but there are a variety of options.

Remember, if mom is nursing, the rash will also be on her nipples if it is in baby's mouth. She needs to be treated too so that mom and baby don't pass the infection back and forth.

If the rash is in the diaper area, and baby is in cloth diapers, then the diapers need to be thoroughly washed and stripped. Disposables may be used temporarily to help the rash clear up while the diapers are being washed. They can even be boiled to completely kill the yeast (check the manufacturer's directions). Add tea tree oil to the wash and Dawn dish soap and rinse in hot water several times. Cloth diapers can harbor yeast and re-infect the baby if they are not cleaned.

- **Probiotics** – Fighting the yeast back into balance by getting good bacteria into the body is key. Probiotic powders and supplements should be offered to the baby/child orally. Older children can consume probiotic foods. Klaire Labs makes a powder for infants (allergy-free).

- **Yogurt** – Used for the probiotics, this can be spread on a yeast rash in the diaper area to combat it directly.
- **Coconut oil** – This is anti-fungal and can help to fight the yeast rash.
- **Tea tree oil** – This should be very diluted, but it is also anti-fungal and can help to combat the rash.
- **Genetian Violet** – If nothing else is working, this can be used on an oral yeast rash. It is typically very effective.

FOOD ALLERGIES

In addition to eczema, food allergies can cause rashes like:

- Red, itchy ring around the mouth
- Red ring around the anus
- Hives
- Red, patchy rash on the cheeks
- Dark circles around the eyes

Any rash which shows up soon after consuming food or which seems to be constant (i.e. not attributable to an acute illness) should be considered as a possible food or other allergy reaction. Talk to an alternative doctor and consider an elimination diet. Of the rashes above, hives would be the most serious – it shows the possibility of an IgE or IgG reaction, and the next time the child consumes that food, anaphylactic shock could result. Be very careful with hives and seek allergy testing if you are unsure what has caused them.

Any suspicious, unusual rash should be shown to a medical professional for diagnosis. Once it has been identified, it can possibly be treated at home with any of the above remedies. If a rash is accompanied by any serious symptoms (trouble breathing, unresponsive behavior, lethargy, etc.) seek medical help immediately.

During the warm months – whether that's just a few per year or most of the year, depending on your location – outdoor play is common and should be encouraged. However, this means that sunburns, bugs, and other "outdoor specific" issues crop up. The mainstream sunscreens, burn lotions, and bug sprays aren't safe for skin. Sunscreens also block the very important UVB rays, which are responsible for producing vitamin D in the skin.

On the issue of sunscreens, ideally, they should be skipped as often as possible. Children need vitamin D and the absolute best place to get it is the sun[228]. How much sun is required depends on the location, time of year, how much skin is exposed, and how fair the skin tone is. Water interferes with the development of vitamin D in the skin.

The UVB rays are strongest around mid-day[229]. Earlier and later in the day, UVA rays (which are responsible for most of the skin damage, including skin cancers) are stronger and more prevalent in the earlier and later parts of the day. Therefore, children should receive their sun exposure at mid-day if at all possible – as close to solar "noon" as possible (which is 1 PM during daylight savings time). They should wear as little clothing as they can. Children who are at higher latitudes, in areas where it is cold in the winter, cannot get enough vitamin D between September and March (fall and winter months) even if it is sunny.

Many sunscreens contain nanoparticles, which may penetrate the skin and get into the bloodstream – research is currently uncertain on this point[230]. Others contain a lot of "extra" ingredients that are simply unsafe[231]. Finally, sunburn can often be avoided by consuming foods rich in saturated fats, making sure vitamin D levels are optimized[232], and avoiding polyunsaturated fats. Processed foods in general increase the likelihood of sunburn, and real foods decrease the risk[233].

My own children don't wear sunscreen at all. Even in the middle of the summer, even if they are out all day, even though they are extremely fair. They don't burn. None have ever had a sunburn. There have been occasions that *I* have burned slightly, but they have not. A healthy diet strongly affects whether or not one burns.

Some parents still feel that their children need sunscreen, at least sometimes. Perhaps they live in very hot climates or are outdoors many hours a day. Perhaps their diet isn't yet optimal and they can't rely on full protection there. Some kids are prone to burns. Others are prone to bugs (consuming a lot of sugar seems to increase this). There are safe ways to keep kids from burns and bugs.

- **Timing** – Avoiding the sun in the mid-morning or late afternoon is a good idea, because this is when the UVA rays are the strongest, and the UVB rays are the weakest. Mid-day sun exposure will maximize vitamin D production and minimize damage to the skin.

228   http://www.scientificamerican.com/article.cfm?id=vitamin-d-deficiency-united-states
229   http://www.sciencedaily.com/releases/2005/05/050526091912.htm
230   http://phys.org/news201517128.html
231   http://www.ewg.org/nanotechnology-sunscreens
232   http://www.nature.com/jid/journal/v125/n5/full/5603599a.html
233   http://www.nature.com/jid/journal/v125/n5/full/5603599a.html

- **Zinc oxide** – This is a safe chemical that provides a physical barrier against the skin. You can buy a zinc-oxide-based cream or buy the zinc oxide to make your own.

- **Coconut oil** – This oil has a slight SPF of about 5. Rubbing it onto skin or using it in a homemade sun block can help to fight off sunburn.

- **Carrot seed oil** – This oil has sun protective qualities, absorbing UV rays.

- **Raspberry oil** – This oil also has sun protective qualities (and is sometimes used in homemade sun blocks).

- **Citronella essential oil** – This essential oil is known for keeping bugs at bay. Mix it with a carrier oil to about 2% dilution and spray it on directly, or put it in a diffuser near a play area.

- **Thyme essential oil** – This essential oil can also help keep bugs at bay. Thyme plants in an area may help to keep bugs away.

- **Rosemary essential oil** – This essential oil can also help keep bugs at bay (used in a homemade bug spray) or rosemary plants in an area may help.

- **Apis** – This is a homeopathic remedy that can help reduce swelling and other reactions to bug bites or stings.

- **Bentonite Clay** – Apply this as a thin paste to any bug bite or sting to help draw out the poison and reduce pain.

- **Aloe vera** – Pure aloe vera (not a lotion that contains it) can help to soothe burned, irritated skin after sun exposure.

Try a combination of the above to meet your needs. Remember not to use any form of sun block too often so that children can get vitamin D from the sun.

If you are not interested in making your own sun block or bug spray, check out the Environmental Working Group's list of safe products[234] to find a commercial option. Badger is a fairly safe brand, as are products made by Made On Hard Lotion.

Poison ivy, oak, and other similar conditions are also "outdoor" issues. Please see the section on Skin Rashes for more on these.

---

234   http://breakingnews.ewg.org/2012sunscreen/

Chicken Pox

This is now an uncommon ailment because so many children are vaccinated for it. It used to be something everyone got, and most of today's parents, who were born before the vaccine was in wide-spread use (it came out in 1995) have had it. It causes a fever, lethargy, and lack of appetite, followed by an outbreak of red blisters that are very itchy and filled with pus. The blisters last about a week before they scab over and it is done.

While the blisters are erupting (which happens in crops over a few days) the person is very contagious. They are also contagious just before the spots erupt. While the chicken pox makes an itchy and uncomfortable week for many children, they recover from it with no issues. There are ways to make the child more comfortable during the rash, though.

- **Baking Soda** – Add this to a warm bath to soothe the itching of the pox.
- **Oatmeal** – Add this (or use oatstraw) to a warm bath to soothe the itching too.
- **Anti-viral lotion** – A lotion containing coconut oil, avocado oil, and rosemary oil may help combat the itching and heal the spots faster. (Avocado oil is nourishing to make up for the drying nature of coconut oil.)
- **Oregano oil** – This is a potent anti-viral essential oil, which can be diluted and used topically. Certain brands can also be taken internally, but check carefully with the company or distributor for instructions.
- **Garlic** – This is a potent anti-viral. Crush it and swallow it, covered in honey. For smaller children, a tiny amount of crushed garlic can be added to a bowl of soup (warm, not hot).
- **Mullein** – This is an herb which is nourishing and anti-viral. It could be infused into a lotion, or taken as a tea.

Rubella

For young children, rubella is typically a very mild illness. It usually produces a low fever for a few days (along with lack of appetite, some fussiness, tiredness), followed by a red rash. It's similar to roseola, but usually milder, and causes no lasting issues. It may also cause cold-like symptoms: runny nose, cough, swollen lymph nodes. The rash typically starts on or around the face and moves downwards. The whole illness typically lasts 2 – 4 days in younger kids (under 10). It is really only dangerous in pregnant women, when it can cause Congenital Rubella Syndrome (it crosses the placenta to infect the unborn baby), but this only occurs earlier in pregnancy.

Most measures are comfort/support-related.

- **Rest** – Most children will be fairly tired for the first couple of days, so let them rest as needed.
- **Mullein** – This anti-viral herb may help to support the immune system and help the virus runs its course more quickly and easily. Offer as a tea.
- **Warm baths** – These should help the child relax and hopefully sleep. As long as they can rest, just leave them alone.

- **Ginger** – This can be used as a tea to help any respiratory symptoms or sore throat.
- **Peppermint** – As an oil, diluted, this can be used to combat a headache, if one develops (more common in older children/adults).

Meningitis

This one *really* scares parents, and it can be truly serious. Most people who experience any symptoms of meningitis do need to be seen by a medical professional immediately. Bacterial meningitis is more serious than viral. Symptoms include fever, severe, headache, stiff neck, vomiting, confusion, and seizures. In some cases, people experience skin rashes, dizziness, or sensitivity to light. Sometimes very young children do not display typical symptoms and instead have a shrill cry (especially when being carried/moved) or have trouble breathing[235].

If you suspect meningitis, seek a doctor's diagnosis. Bacterial meningitis needs to be treated quickly and may require antibiotics. Viral meningitis, which is milder, can often be managed at home – but needs a diagnosis first, so that bacterial meningitis is ruled out. Viral meningitis usually lasts about 3 days (when the person feels fairly ill) and is completely over within 2 weeks. Swelling in the brain/ears may result in deafness, so anti-inflammatory herbs should be used if needed, and a doctor called if they are not working fairly quickly. Home treatment options include:

- **Fluids** – Dehydration is a possibility, so keeping up with fluids is important. Try the electrolyte drink recipe mentioned in the Stomach Viruses section to help prevent dehydration.
- **Garlic** – An anti-viral herb, this can be mixed with coconut oil and put on the feet. Crushed garlic can also be swallowed.
- **Ginger** – This is anti-inflammatory and may help reduce symptoms, especially sore throat and headache.
- **Rest** – A lot of rest is needed for recovery, so rest/sleep should be allowed as desired.
- **Peppermint** – This can reduce the headache that is common with meningitis. Try using the essential oil topically.
- **Lavender** – This essential oil can also reduce headaches, when used topically.
- **Devil's claw** – This herb is a mild pain reliever. A tincture can be used to relieve headache.
- **Arnica** – Used topically as a cream, or homeopathically orally, it can help to relieve muscle aches and pain.

If these remedies are not working within a few days, or more serious symptoms develop, call a doctor immediately. These remedies should *not* be attempted unless meningitis is mild and has been declared viral by a doctor. You may also choose to seek the advice of an alternative doctor.

Mumps

This is another one that can scare parents, because it is said to cause deafness and

---

235   http://children.webmd.com/vaccines/tc/meningitis-symptoms

sterility. While these are *possible* outcomes, they are extremely unlikely. Sterility can only occur in post-pubertal males. Younger children are not at risk for this complication. Even in older males, the infection has to move from its usual location, the salivary glands, to the testes, and it must affect both, in order to have a chance to cause lasting damage. Only 1 in several thousand will experience permanent fertility issues.

Hearing loss, the other concern, occurs in only about 1 in 15,000 cases of mumps[236]. Most cases are fairly mild, worst in teens. Very young children may experience subclinical illness that mimic respiratory illness more than anything else. Typically, the symptoms are fever, fatigue, lack of appetite, pain in the sinuses and jaw, and headache. After a couple of days, swelling occurs in the salivary glands, usually the parotid glands, which gives the characteristic "chipmunk cheek" look. This swelling often occurs on the other side, but not always. It goes down in 2 – 4 days. The entire illness can last a few days to a couple weeks, depending on the age of the person.

There are various home remedies to make the person more comfortable:

- **Rest** – Allow the person to rest as much as possible to help heal, as with any illness.
- **Ginger** – Try some ginger tea or capsules as an anti-inflammatory, to reduce swelling and pain.
- **Bland foods** – Strong or sour foods increase the production of saliva and will hurt someone with mumps due to inflamed salivary glands. Avoid these.
- **Warm/cold compresses** – Depending on the person's preference, compresses that are warm or cold can be used to reduce the swelling in the salivary glands.
- **Belladonna** – This is a homeopathic remedy commonly used for mumps. However, it is not the only option, so talk to a qualified homeopath to find the appropriate remedy in your situation.
- **Mullein** – This is especially beneficial for viral infections as well as respiratory infections, and when combined with catnip, is supposed to be very effective against mumps.

If any complications develop, call a doctor. In most cases the illness will heal without incident, especially in younger children.

Measles

This worries parents because of a risk of complications up to and including death. It can also cause blindness. However, this particular complication is associated with vitamin A deficiency[237]. In most cases, measles is an acute illness with no lasting effects.

Typically, measles starts out with headache, fever, cough, light sensitivity, and muscle pain. After a few days, the rash develops, starting at the head and moving down. At first the rash is flat, and slowly becomes raised bumps. It takes 1 – 2 weeks to heal from measles in most cases. There is no specific treatment for it and home/supportive care is

---

236   http://www.virology-online.com/viruses/MUMPS.htm
237   http://www.ncbi.nlm.nih.gov/pubmed/14998696

usually all that is needed.

- **Rest** – As with any illness, allow rest as needed.
- **Mullein** – Serve as a tea to combat the virus.
- **FCLO** -- This contains vitamin A and D to help prevent complications and boost the immune system.
- **Warm baths** – To help the child relax if needed.
- **Anti-viral lotion** – To help calm the rash, especially if itchy.

If the child shows any signs of complications, which are very rare but potentially serious, call a health professional.

Pertussis

This infection is actually epidemic currently in many parts of the country, in both vaccinated and unvaccinated individuals. It is referred to as "the 100 day cough" because of its length and severity. While older children and adults can experience pertussis as little more than an unusually long respiratory infection, young babies are at serious risk. The thickened mucus and inability to clear it (the pertussis bacteria paralyzes the cilia in the lungs so that clearing the thick mucus produced is difficult – hence the strong cough and eventual "whoop" of indrawn breath) mean that babies may struggle to breathe and even require hospitalization. Very young babies can even die from it.

Pertussis typically starts out as a normal cold – runny nose, sneezing, sore throat, maybe a mild cough. As the cold symptoms begin to ease, the cough gets worse. It may be difficult for the person to catch their breath. It may lead to intense coughing fits, especially at night, which can cause vomiting. The person will cough up the thickened mucus eventually, although this is difficult due to the pertussis bacteria. In severe cases, hospitalization for supportive care (oxygen, suctioning) may be required. Most older children and adults (by age 1 – 2) can treat this at home.

There are several effective home treatments.

- **Vitamin C** – Probably the best treatment is high-dose vitamin C. Children are given up to 5000mg per day, consistently, which often lessens the cough so that it is still present but not so severe. It must be kept up for weeks until the infection is over. Acerola powder (pure) is one natural source of vitamin C.
- **Fluids** – Staying hydrated is important because it can help to thin the mucus a bit, making it easier to cough up.
- **Zinc** – This supplement may help to boost the immune system and is recommended by our pediatrician at the onset of any illness. It has been shown to have some benefit in respiratory illnesses.
- **FCLO** – Cod liver oil, with its high levels of vitamins A and D can help to boost the immune system and clear the body of excess mucus.
- **Mullein** – When combined with coltsfoot (another herb), it can help get the mucus out of the body more effectively. These can be taken as a tea or a syrup.
- **Slippery elm** – This is another herb that may increase mucus production as well as

thinning it. Serve as a tea with lemon and honey (if the child is over a year).

- **Humidifier** – Use a humidifier to keep the child's nasal passages moist, especially during sleep. Some do better with cool air rather than warm air, and at certain times of year, an open window may be helpful.

If the child struggles to breathe or is breathing shallowly or rapidly, or if the lips turn blue or the child is unable to catch their breath – seek medical attention. In a young baby, seek medical attention immediately. With the above treatments, most older children will recover and will not need additional help. The cough can last for months and may leave the child more vulnerable to further infections for awhile. Continue to boost the child's immune system with FCLO and a healthy diet to try to prevent infections, and avoid crowds during the winter and early spring months.

While all of these illnesses can be scary, arming yourself with information is key. Don't listen to the scare tactics like "Your child will die!" or "Your child will be deaf or blind!" Learn what each illness is really like and what the chances of complications really are (minimal). Then, learn to treat them at home when possible, and when to call the doctor. These illnesses are "mysterious" because many of us have never seen them and that is why they scare us. But they don't have to – learn about them now so that if your child should ever experience them, you're armed with the information you need to navigate them calmly and with common sense.

FOOD ALLERGIES

Food allergies are becoming increasingly more common[238]. When most of today's parents were growing up in the 80s and 90s, food allergies were almost unheard of. Perhaps they would run across a child with an allergy here or there, but it was not very often (I personally heard of perhaps 2 – 3 children who had allergies the entire time I was growing up).

These days, however, *many* children have some form of food allergy[239] or intolerance[240]. It is common for children to be dairy-free, gluten-free, nut-free, and all kinds of other "free." There are now dedicated nut-free tables in school cafeterias, and some schools are completely free of nuts. (Not one of those kids I knew growing up had a nut allergy.)

For some reason, parents haven't questioned this. It just "is what it is" and kids have a lot of allergies for "some unknown reason." Parents studiously learn what foods need to be avoided and then do so. There are even entire websites dedicated to finding both recipes and packaged food items that are "free" of common allergens. All packaged foods are required by law to be labeled which of the top 7 allergens they contain. Food allergies are big.

The top 7 allergens are:

- Tree Nuts
- Peanuts
- Soy
- Dairy
- Gluten
- Seafood
- Eggs

These are responsible for the majority of allergies. However, corn (which is gluten-free) is becoming increasingly common. Children are also cross-reacting to plants in the same family now. Latex allergies may result in sensitivities to mango and avocado. Nightshade sensitivities include tomatoes, peppers, eggplants, and potatoes. Severe nut allergies may also include coconut, which is not technically a nut. Severe peanut allergies could result in other legume allergies (peas, beans).

The top two allergens (by number of children who suffer) are dairy and soy. The most severe allergies are usually caused by peanuts or tree nuts. Of course, a child can be allergic to *anything* – any fruit, vegetable, grain, etc. no matter how common or uncommon it is. It's almost harder with an uncommon allergen because they're not labeled. Plus, products may contain "hidden" sources of even common allergens, so parents have to become savvy to labeling tricks. Even worse, some products labeled as being "free" of an allergen might contain trace amounts or become cross-contaminated in certain facilities, so those with allergies must be even more careful. Most with

---

238   http://www.cnn.com/2011/HEALTH/06/20/food.allergies.pediatrics/index.html
239   http://pediatrics.aappublications.org/content/130/1/e25.full
240   http://today.msnbc.msn.com/id/43447764/ns/today-today_health/t/peanuts-milk-shellfish-kids-may-have-food-allergies#.UNOmHuRJOAg

severe allergies can't eat in restaurants or away from home at all for fear of cross-contamination.

Food allergies are likely caused by a number of factors, but the biggest factor is gut health[241], [242]. Most people these days consume a lot of processed foods, which can damage the gut. They also don't consume fermented foods, so their gut flora is poor and their gut may become "leaky," meaning that their guts have "holes" where there is no good gut flora, which allows undigested proteins to seep into the bloodstream. These proteins are treated as foreign invaders and the body attacks them – causing an allergy to that food. Pesticides in tap water, which can also affect the gut, has also been implicated in the development of food allergies[243].

Leaky gut has also been blamed for autoimmune disorders[244], Crohn's disease[245], celiac disease, chronic fatigue syndrome[246], depression[247], and more.

This can happen in a mother, which sensitizes her baby's gut before birth. New research shows that babies aren't born with sterile guts[248], but are in fact building up gut flora in the womb as they are swallowing the amniotic fluid from mid-pregnancy[249]. The "stuff" they swallow either passes out of the baby as urine in the womb, or it is stored up in the intestines as meconium. This meconium is the beginning of the baby's gut flora. The baby also gains more gut flora during the passage through the birth canal.

After birth, baby's gut flora continues to build from sucking on his hands, breathing, nursing (or bottle feeding) and so on. If mom has a leaky gut and is nursing, she can pass undigested proteins to her baby, sensitizing the baby, who is born with a naturally leaky gut. The IgA in breastmilk helps to mature the gut[250], [251] and "seal" it over time (babies who are formula-fed from birth have delayed gut maturation and may never fully normally mature; elective c-sections are also a problem[252]). Unfortunately, most formulas contain a lot of corn, soy, and milk, which is likely part of the reason these allergies are now so common.

Since some evidence shows that proper gut maturation is critical for correct immune function[253], gut health is a big deal!

What To Do About Food Allergies

In a perfect world, if a mother had some health concerns or known food sensitivities, she would address these prior to becoming pregnant. Although there are many reasons why a woman chooses to get pregnant when she does (age, child spacing, etc.), the best way to avoid a child with food allergies is to heal the mother's gut before conceiving.

241   http://www.cnn.com/2010/HEALTH/08/03/food.allergies.er.gut/index.html
242   http://www.ncbi.nlm.nih.gov/pubmed/10480760
243   http://abcnews.go.com/m/blogEntry?id=17866028
244   http://www.ncbi.nlm.nih.gov/pubmed/22109896
245   http://www.ncbi.nlm.nih.gov/pubmed/10980980
246   http://www.ncbi.nlm.nih.gov/pubmed/19112401
247   http://www.ncbi.nlm.nih.gov/pubmed/18283240
248   http://syontix.com/what-are-beneficial-gut-flora/
249   http://www.ncbi.nlm.nih.gov/pubmed/18330727
250   http://www.ncbi.nlm.nih.gov/pubmed/18330727
251   http://www.ncbi.nlm.nih.gov/pubmed/17596738
252   http://ajpregu.physiology.org/content/294/3/R929.full
253   http://www.ncbi.nlm.nih.gov/pubmed/22726443

This is not an easy or quick task, which is why many women feel overwhelmed and choose not to go this route. A woman may need six months to two years to do something called the GAPS diet before they are healed enough to get rid of their own food allergies and other health concerns. After they transition off the diet, they should eat a well-balanced, nourishing, traditional diet for six months, and then attempt conception. So, obviously, a woman who chooses to heal herself first is putting off having a baby by one to three years. Still, this is ideal and women who have serious health concerns should consider this. This book is not about pre-conception or pregnancy so it will not go in-depth on this issue.

Once a child with food allergies has been born, what then? Gut health can be addressed in the child also using a GAPS protocol, ideally as young as possible. If food allergies are discovered in the early months, the child should be exclusively breastfed while the mother begins the GAPS diet, and no solid foods should be introduced until healing has began. Early foods should be bone broths, meat, and probiotic foods (yogurt, if there is no dairy issue). Nuts, grains, soy, vegetables, and anything the mom or baby is still reacting to should be avoided.

Older children can also recover, by removing the allergens from their diet and beginning GAPS. It is not an easy diet to follow and many parents feel at a loss – "But GAPS eliminates the only foods he will actually eat!" This is usually the case because the pathogenic gut flora prefers grains, sugar, fruit, and often dairy products. I have personally gone through this with my own daughter and she only liked those foods...and we managed to do GAPS anyway. It is a transition, it can be difficult, but there are ways to make it through. See my articles online[254] about our experiences with GAPS for more.

The bottom line? Children do not have to just "deal with it" for the rest of their lives. There are ways to heal the gut and in the process, heal food allergies. Read the GAPS book by Dr. Natasha Campbell-McBride for more information.

I also encourage families whose children are suffering from food allergies to avoid processed foods, even "safe" ones. The food additives included in those items will not help the gut to heal and could prolong healing or cause further damage.

Many in the mainstream, especially doctors, will tell you that healing food allergies is impossible. That is not true. Most doctors do not believe the "leaky gut" theory. However, an increasing number of doctors, both "alternative" and "mainstream" (holistic-leaning) doctors are beginning to believe in this theory and see the changes that GAPS can have.

If you or your child has severe food allergies, especially multiple issues or anaphylactic reactions, please find a qualified GAPS physician[255] under whom to begin this program. They are out there, and they are necessary for those with serious health concerns. You may also choose to seek one out if you are not sure what issues your child has and if your child could benefit from the GAPS protocol or not.

254   http://www.modernalternativemama.com/gaps-and-grain-free/
255   http://gaps.me/preview/?page_id=496

SEASONAL ALLERGIES

Seasonal allergies are another major and increasing concern that parents have. And with good reason – these, too, are on the rise.

Many children (and adults) find themselves with watery eyes, sneezing, coughing, and more during spring and fall. They're concerned about pollen counts, need to avoid the outdoors at certain times, keep windows closed, and run special air filters in their homes. This becomes miserable, and the normal course of action is to keep a very clean home and take over-the-counter or prescription antihistamines.

Are there other ways to deal with seasonal allergies? Yes. See the previous section on food allergies – many seasonal allergies are rooted in the gut, and a GAPS protocol could help to heal them. GAPS is used less frequently for seasonal allergies than food allergies because of the less-obvious connection, but there have been reports of those who have been helped.

Another option is something called "NAET," which is a muscle-energy method of realigning the body and clearing it of allergens. I am unsure how effective this is long-term and if it really addresses the underlying causes, but there have been reports of people who have been helped by it.

There are additional options as well, which are easier, less expensive, and more readily available. There is some scientific evidence that some of these may be used instead of or in conjunction with conventional therapies[256].

- **Freeze-Dried Nettles** – Many swear by capsules of this herb, which contains a natural anti-histamine. For some reason, the nettles need to be freeze-dried to be effective.

- **Local Raw Honey** – It must be *local*, within an hour's drive. The raw honey contains pollen and other "allergens" that gently helps the body to overcome the reaction.

- **Quercetin** – This is a natural compound found in various fruits and vegetables and it appears to combat allergies in some.

- **Vitamin C** – This, too, may boost the body's ability to fight off an allergic reaction.

- **Bromelain** – A natural enzyme found in pineapple (especially in the core), this may help seasonal allergies.

- **Chinese Medicine** – There are various herbal preparations that claim to reduce symptoms. Trilight Health is a company that makes one version and several readers I've spoken to have found it helps quite a bit. There is some scientific evidence that blends like these may help[257].

- **Neti Pot** – The use of a neti pot (with filtered water, not tap) can help to rinse out the sinuses and reduce the symptoms associated with seasonal allergies.

Others swear by certain essential oils (frankincense is common) or other remedies. Experiment to see which remedy(ies) work best for you.

---

256   http://www.ncbi.nlm.nih.gov/pubmed/11056414
257   http://www.ncbi.nlm.nih.gov/pubmed/14526714

Many parents wonder how they can keep their child's teeth clean and strong. The mainstream dentists recommend brushing a child's teeth as soon as they come in, as well as giving oral fluoride, having regular cleanings, topical fluoride, and dental sealants. These are not the safest ways to keep a child's teeth healthy.

Fluoride has not been shown to be effective at preventing tooth decay either orally or topically[258]. It also can cause fluorosis in large doses[259] and may be toxic to the body[260].

Dental sealants contain BPA, an endocrine disruptor[261]. "Amalgam" fillings and "silver" fillings contain mercury. These have not been shown to be safe, and in fact, the mercury may lead to toxicity issues[262].

What's a concerned parent to do?

Diet has a major impact on dental health. As most know, consuming too much sugar has a negative impact on the teeth. The large consumption of refined flours and sugars induces dental decay[263]. On the other hand, vitamin K2, which is found in pastured dairy products and a few other animal sources, has been shown to combat it[264].

A child's palate (the shape of his/her jaw and mouth) is affected by nutrition. A well-nourished mother will produce a child with a wider palate that has plenty of space for all 32 adult teeth. However, it is possible to affect a child's palate later in life (during childhood, and sometimes even during adulthood – anecdotally) by feeding them nourishing foods like butter oil[265].

Breastfeeding is also an important part of palate development[266]. Breastmilk contains the nutrients a child needs to grow strong bones and teeth[267]. It also doesn't contain the same sugars as cow's milk or formula and doesn't contribute to tooth decay[268]. Plus, the physical act of breastfeeding (the position of the baby in relation to the mom's breast and the position of the nipple in his/her mouth) contributes to overall development as well[269]. Children breastfed at least 6 months had a lowered risk of oral development issues; children who were bottle-fed for a year had 10 times the risk of oral development issues[270]. The longer a child was breastfed, the lower their risk of oral development problems. Breastfeeding until age 2 or 3, when all of a child's baby teeth are in can help proper oral development.

Choosing a safer toothpaste is a good idea. It should not contain fluoride, for the

258   http://articles.mercola.com/sites/articles/archive/2012/01/03/fluoride-show-no-benefits.aspx
259   http://articles.mercola.com/sites/articles/archive/2012/01/03/fluoride-show-no-benefits.aspx
260   http://articles.mercola.com/sites/articles/archive/2012/01/03/fluoride-show-no-benefits.aspx
261   http://articles.mercola.com/sites/articles/archive/2012/01/03/fluoride-show-no-benefits.aspx
262   http://articles.mercola.com/sites/articles/archive/2012/04/07/dangers-of-mercury-contamination.aspx
263   http://wholehealthsource.blogspot.com/2009/01/tokelau-island-migrant-study-dental.html
264   http://www.healingteethnaturally.com/vitamin-k2-dr-weston-price-activator-x.html
265   http://www.cheeseslave.com/can-good-nutrition-widen-a-childs-palate-even-after-birth/
266   http://www.ncbi.nlm.nih.gov/pubmed/2656791
267   http://www.jaoa.org/content/106/4/203.full
268   http://milkmatters.org.uk/2010/12/05/breastfeeding-tooth-decay/
269   http://www.brianpalmerdds.com/bfeed_oralcavity.htm
270   http://www.jped.com.br/conteudo/03-79-01-07/ing.pdf

reasons stated previously. It also should not contain glycerin, which may affect tooth remineralization[271]. One brand is Earthpaste, which is made from a base of bentonite clay. It has the advantage of being gentler on tooth enamel and gums than baking soda (upon which many natural toothpastes are based) and it doesn't contain glycerin or other questionable ingredients. It is safe to swallow, so small children can use it. Children only need to brush gently, with a very soft-bristled toothbrush.

Some children do not brush at all. Plaque is formed from bacteria, saliva, proteins, sugars, and fats. Only certain types of bacteria are capable of causing tooth decay. These bacteria largely feed on simple sugars, which are so prevalent in the modern diet[272]. Fermented foods for healthier gut flora and consuming few simple sugars and starches sharply lowers the risk of tooth decay and plaque, so young children with a healthy diet may or may not need to brush.

Older children (over 7 or 8) may choose to explore an alternate method of oral health, oil pulling. Oil pulling involves using a small amount of healthy oil in the mouth (sesame or coconut, most often) to swish very gently for about 10 minutes. This oil cleans the teeth and gums, pulling any toxins out of the very sensitive oral cavity. The oil will become mixed with saliva and will be very thin, sometimes grayish, and fairly "gross" by the end of the swishing time.

Oil pulling is best done on an empty stomach (first thing in the morning) and the mouth should be rinsed thoroughly with clean water afterward. Only children who are old enough not to swallow can do this – the oil will be full of bacteria and should not be swallowed; doing so is unhealthy. About one teaspoon of oil is enough for an 8 – 12 year old; a teen or adult can use up to 1 tablespoon. Oil pulling has been shown to be effective in reducing the bacteria that is primarily responsible for tooth decay[273].

With a focus on proper diet (nutrient-dense foods with very little refined grain or sugar), the teeth will develop healthy and strong. There is some evidence that supplementing with raw butter oil can help heal tooth decay[274], should it occur. The book *Cure Tooth Decay* has more details. Should a child have this issue, especially in baby teeth, natural methods of healing are preferable to fillings.

Although root canals are typically performed on adults, they may also be recommended for children (in order to "keep the spacing" for when the permanent teeth come in later). They are dangerous, however, and have been linked to cancer, among other issues[275]. Removing the tooth if it cannot be saved is preferable.

What about annual x-rays? In most cases, they are not really needed. If a child has a suspected problem, they may be warranted in that case. Annual x-rays have been shown to increase the risk of brain tumors[276]. Typical aprons shield the body, but not the neck, and this increases the risk of thyroid disorders, including thyroid cancer[277]. X-rays should be used only where needed, and children should wear a full apron,

271   http://community.curetoothdecay.com/cavities/topics/glycerine_stops_teeth_from_repairing
272   http://www.adha.org/CE_courses/course7/plaque_formation.htm
273   http://www.ncbi.nlm.nih.gov/pubmed/18408265
274   http://www.curetoothdecay.com/Baby_Bottle_Tooth_Decay/fermented-cod-liver-butter-oil-green-pasture-baby-cavities.htm
275   http://www.westonaprice.org/dentistry/root-canal-dangers
276   http://www.cbsnews.com/8301-504763_162-57411765-10391704/yearly-dental-x-rays-raise-brain-tumor-risk-study-finds/
277   http://worldental.org/dental-news/thyroid-cancer-risks-increased-by-dental-x-rays/1289/

including a thyroid guard, if they are receiving them.

Seek a holistic dentist if possible in your area. A holistic dentist will not push drilling, filling, and fluoride treatments, and will be informed about the link between nutrition and dental health.

Challenge the traditional dental paradigm, but be smart: if your child has an infection, is in pain, has obvious tooth decay, or another issue – go see a dentist. Dentists are there if they are needed.

My own children rarely brush their teeth. We focus on healthy diet and supplementing with FCLO/BO. They all have straight, white, uncrowded teeth and wide jaws (despite my own very narrow jaw). As long as this continues, we'll keep going on the path that we are. At this time, only one child has seen a dentist, for a suspected infection (the child claimed "my teeth hurt" but later it became evident that there was an infection in the lymph nodes surrounding the jaw, not the teeth) and the dentist said all the teeth were perfect, no issues. When they do brush – which they enjoy – they use Earthpaste. It is possible to have healthy teeth and gums using alternative methods!

One of the most common concerns that parents have about their children is sleep. Are they getting enough of it? Are they sleeping in long enough stretches? Are they sleeping similarly to their peers? How can they be 'taught' to sleep independently? Of course, since a child's sleep patterns directly affect their parent's, and sleep-deprived parents struggle, there is good reason for the concern with sleep.

Normal Baby Sleep

Normal babies spend the first three to four months sleeping and waking somewhat randomly around the clock. They sleep in 2 – 4 hour stretches and then are awake for an hour or two. They also sleep very lightly so that they will easily wake due to hunger. This is *normal*, not a problem, and will slowly change so that most sleep is done at night, with 2 – 3 "naps" throughout the day.

Although our culture has come to believe that babies ought to sleep through the night by 6 weeks of age, the actual age at which most children truly sleep through the night is closer to two or three *years* old, and some children up to age 2 were found to wake an average of 2.5 times per night[278]. Parents whose babies are still waking every 2 – 3 hours to eat when they are 6, 8, 10 months old are not alone[279].

Babies cannot be "taught" to sleep by ignoring their cries[280]. Babies cry to communicate, and it is the only means they have[281] Babies continue to have a need for comfort, warmth, food, and many other things throughout the first year or two. Some are very bothered by teething, illness, or a wet diaper. Babies who are fitful or sleep poorly need a parent who can figure out what the issue is – there is some sort of discomfort there. Some babies sleep poorly due to undiscovered food allergies. Others are sensitive to temperature changes or the texture of clothing or their sheets.

Over time, babies will learn to sleep in longer stretches and will need less attention at night. It takes much longer than many parents think, but all babies eventually get there.

With both of my boys, feeding them extra throughout the day and especially before bed was helpful. They would wake at 9 – 12 months because they were growing rapidly and they were hungry. When they were offered enough nourishing food throughout the day, they slept better – eggs, butter, avocado, fatty meats, etc. We also offered them plain yogurt and/or a banana as a bed time snack. This is fine for older babies or toddlers. It should not be attempted with younger babies, who are still meant to wake to eat.

Teething may also present an issue with sleep. Our best solution was to offer a "teething tea" immediately before bed. This consisted of ½ c. water, 1 tsp. catnip, and 4 – 5 whole cloves, boiled and lightly sweetened with maple syrup or honey. There are also teething creams[282], amber teething necklaces (they are not to be chewed on; the succinic acid in the amber absorbs into the skin and provides some pain relief), homeopathic teething tablets, and other remedies. We found the teething tea to be the safest and

278   http://www.ncbi.nlm.nih.gov/pubmed/21784676
279   http://www.ncbi.nlm.nih.gov/pubmed/21784676
280   http://www.askdrsears.com/topics/fussy-baby/science-says-excessive-crying-could-be-harmful
281   http://www.psychologytoday.com/blog/moral-landscapes/201112/dangers-crying-it-out
282   http://www.modernalternativemama.com/blog/2012/02/27/monday-health-wellness-home-made-teething-cream/

most effective. One of our babies had a reaction to the teething tablets in the form of insomnia, which was most definitely not helpful!

Finally, all our older children (starting around a year) take a cup of plain water to bed with them. Water alone is safe as it won't cause dental issues. Also, they do not hold and suck on the cup constantly; they wake briefly, take a drink, and go back to sleep. If the cup is in their beds, they will take a quick drink and resettle themselves. If not, they will cry until we bring them a drink.

Sleep Issues in Older Kids

Many parents struggle with bedtime. Their kids don't want to go to bed, and bedtime becomes a long, drawn-out process.

The problems with sleep could be any number of things. There is little research exploring the cause of sleep problems, but the resulting issues (bedtime struggles, insomnia, snoring) have been linked to problems like ADHD and learning disabilities later in childhood[283].

One possible reason for sleep disturbances is allergies or poor gut health. Reflux can also cause an issue[284]. Poor sleep usually does have a physical cause of some sort, but unfortunately there is very little research in this area right now. Most of the evidence is anecdotal.

Magnesium deficiency can affect sleep. Magnesium helps promote restful sleep and insomnia is one of the early signs of deficiency[285]. Adults who use a magnesium supplement topically and sometimes orally usually experience increased ability to fall asleep and stay asleep throughout the night; such supplementation is usually safe for toddlers and beyond (check with a doctor in your child's case to be sure). Restless legs that prevent sleep is usually a sign to use magnesium or possibly potassium.

There is some evidence that B12[286] or D deficiencies could be related to sleep issues, especially night terrors. Most mainstream doctors write night terrors off as "due to emotional stress" and state that children will eventually outgrow them. They are little help in solving this issue, so parents whose children experience them may need to experiment with some supplements. The help of an alternative or holistic doctor may prove valuable in this case. It is known, however, that about 10% of children who undergo general anesthesia will experience night terrors[287], so this may be a cause for a small number of children.

Bed wetting, another common concern, may be linked to several different things. It is associated with ADHD[288] (which is often caused by poor gut health and/or vitamin D deficiency, suggesting that bedwetting may be linked to these as well). Food allergies, especially milk and sometimes gluten, may increase the risk of bedwetting[289]. Dietary changes, elimination diets, and supplements (if needed) may help stop bedwetting.

283 http://www.huffingtonpost.com/2012/09/23/children-sleep-problems-linked-special-education_n_1891081.html
284 http://www.ncbi.nlm.nih.gov/pmc/articles/PMC3485348/
285 http://www.ncbi.nlm.nih.gov/pubmed/21226679
286 http://forums.bettermedicine.com/showthread.php/88477-Hashimoto-and-B12
287 http://www.webmd.com/sleep-disorders/night-terrors
288 http://www.sciencedaily.com/releases/2002/10/021022071217.htm
289 http://bedwettingchildren.com/food-allergies-and-bedwetting/

Sometimes, children may not sleep due to pain. For some, a chiropractic adjustment can make a big difference. Seek the advice of a trained pediatric chiropractor if you suspect this is an issue for your child. We have experienced this with one of my sons.

My own daughter woke frequently at night, especially around a year. She would wake and sometimes scream for an hour straight. Ultimately, removing dairy and gluten from her diet proved helpful and she began to wake only once per night for a diaper change, and not every night. Each of my other children has followed this pattern until potty training – one brief waking, a few times a week, for diaper changes. (Barring illness, of course.)

Sleep problems are no fun for anyone. Unfortunately there is very little research in this area, as sleep troubles aren't often discussed or are thought of as "something children grow out of." The most helpful thing to do if your child is experiencing a sleep disturbance is to look into an elimination diet, offer probiotics, and seek the help of an alternative doctor who is well-versed in sleep issues and dietary treatments.

Besides the very common ones already discussed, children may face a number of other acute illnesses throughout childhood. There are some remedies for these as well.

Teething

Teething isn't fun, but every baby goes through it. Some teethe worse than others. OTC medications are the usual "solution" for parents, but for the reasons listed in the OTC section, they're not the best choice – especially not as a first solution. (A few parents do choose to use them as a last resort, and that's a judgment call.) There are several effective natural remedies that are also very safe.

- **Teething tablets** – These are a homeopathic combination remedy made by Hyland's. Many parents swear by them. They are generally safe and cause no side effects in most babies, and they dissolve instantly. The remedies contained within are intended to reduce swelling, redness, gum pain and aid sleep. One of our children reacted with insomnia and some children are allergic to the lactose base that they are made from, so they are not suitable for everyone.

- **Teething gel** – There are commercial versions on the market that are rubbed into the gums. They have a mild numbing effect.

- **Teething cream** – A homemade teething cream that contains clove naturally relieves oral pain (and can also be used for older children or adults for oral issues).

- **Amber teething necklace** – An amber necklace is worn around the neck and is not to be chewed on. The amber contains succinic acid, a mild analgesic. It warms when against the skin and absorbs, relieving teething pain in many babies.

- **Teething rings** – A wooden teething ring to bite on is helpful for some babies, as the pressure can relieve some pain.

- **Frozen apple slices** – Apples contain an enzyme that helps relieve pain, and when frozen, the cold can help even more.

- **Cold wash cloth** – A cold wash cloth to bite helps some babies with pain.

Hand, Foot and Mouth Disease

This is also a common childhood illness and especially occurs in children who are in schools or childcare situations, as it spreads rapidly. In 2011, a mutated and more serious strain popped up, and it began to hit more children. It causes fever, headache, loss of appetite, and blisters that appear on the hands, feet, and in the mouth (hence the name). It can cause a lot of pain and last from one week to one month, depending on the person and the severity. Luckily, there are some home remedies to help.

- **Rooibos and lemon balm tea** – These herbs are anti-viral and may help calm the reaction of the body, providing some relief.

- **Garlic** – This is a popular anti-viral food. It can be mixed with coconut oil and put on the feet (which may be too rough on the rash itself) or consumed. Try covering a crushed clove with honey and swallowing, especially for older children or adults.

- **Rosemary** – As an herb, it is anti-viral and antibacterial, and can help prevent secondary infection. Try adding it to soups or other meals.

- **Tea tree oil** – Diluted, it could be incorporated in a lotion and used on the skin (but may be too harsh, especially for small ones). It can also be used in a spray bottle (also diluted) to clean the house to prevent transmission to others.
- For more ideas, please see this post: http://www.modernalternativemama. com/blog/2012/03/31/natural-remedies-for-hand-foot-and-mouth-disease/#. UOHNHuRJOAg

Strep Throat

Many children experience strep throat at some point or another. It causes fever and sore throat with white patches on the throat. In some, it can cause stomach upset or vomiting. This is one that really worries parents, because if it's left untreated, it can turn into scarlet fever and become very serious. Many parents do choose to use antibiotics for it, just in case. There are ways to attempt to treat it at home as well. Contact a doctor if you are worried.

It is probably a good idea to try home remedies for 2 – 3 days and contact a doctor if there is no change or if symptoms worsen at any point.

- **Garlic** – This is anti-viral and a crushed clove should be taken every 4 – 6 hours in the early days on the infection, until symptoms ease.
- **Honey Lemon Pepper** – Mix fresh lemon juice, raw honey, and cayenne pepper and take this solution every 4 – 6 hours. It will clear the sinuses and may help to combat the infection.
- **Ginger** – This can help relieve the pain of sore throat and reduce inflammation. Take in tea form.
- **Goldenseal** – A tincture made from this herb can help prevent the strep bacteria from sticking to the throat tissues. Children need only 4 – 5 drops daily; older children and adults can take up to 15 – 20 drops daily.
- **Echinacea** – This herb can also affect the strep bacteria and should be taken daily for up to two weeks. It should not be used long-term and not by those with an auto-immune condition.
- **Apple cider vinegar** – 1 tsp. to 1 tbsp. ACV (use less for children) should be added to 8 oz. of water and drunk every several hours.
- **Vitamin C** – Take 250 to 500mg every few hours for several days. Try pure acerola powder for a natural source.

Growing Pains

These are achiness that occurs usually in the legs, often at night. They may or may not be related to growing, although are often attributed to such. (I experienced this as a child and still sometimes do, and I am definitely not growing now!) What is often the culprit is a magnesium or potassium deficiency. Using magnesium lotion or having the child eat foods high in potassium (bananas, potatoes) can help in most cases.

Bronchitis

This is a respiratory infection that is fairly common in young children. It causes a cough, fever, body aches, congestion, and sore throat. The cough may be severe and could last up to two weeks. Wheezing may also be present. This is often treated with steroids and breathing treatments, but there are home remedies available too.

- **Mullein and coltsfoot** – These two herbs, when combined, can soothe the cough and get rid of the excess mucus, helping to clear the infection from the body faster. They can also be used separately.
- **Eucalyptus oil** – This essential oil, when used in a humidifier or in any way that produces steam (in a bowl or pot of boiling water, for example) can help to clear breathing passages.
- **Lobelia** – This herb should be used in tincture form and must not be heated. It can help to clear the lungs and ease wheezing.
- **Rest** – As always, rest is essential for healing.
- **FCLO** – Vitamins A and D can help to boost the overall immune system.

Headaches

Everyone experiences a headache now and then. They may be caused by tension, food intolerances, minor injuries, dehydration, sleep deprivation, or just about anything. Most headaches are not serious. Ongoing, severe headaches should be evaluated by a doctor. The average headache can be treated safely and easily at home.

- **Peppermint oil** – This essential oil mixed with a carrier oil can be applied directly to the forehead, temples, or other affected areas to ease headache pain.
- **Arnica** – A salve containing arnica[290] may be used to ease tension headaches.
- **Mullein** – This herb can help ease the pain of migraines. Prepare in a tea or syrup.
- **Massage** – Depending on the cause, massage can help to ease the pain of headaches.
- **Chiropractic** – An adjustment can help ease some headaches, and chiropractors may have additional advice on headache treatments.
- **Avoiding foods** – If you have a known or suspected food allergy or sensitivity, avoiding the trigger food(s) may stop headaches from occurring. Gluten and dairy seem to be triggers for many.
- **Hot compresses** – A rice-filled heating pad placed on the neck or head can help to ease headache pain.
- **Ginger** – This herb is anti-inflammatory and may reduce headache pain.
- **Electrolyte drink** – See the recipe in the Stomach Viruses section. Dehydration can cause headaches and this can help dehydration.

RSV

This is a viral infection similar to the common cold. In most children it is not too serious, but in babies or those who are immune-compromised, it can be. Most children have

---

290   http://www.modernalternativemama.com/blog/2011/12/5/monday-health-wellness-sore-muscle-and-
headache-salve.html

it by age 5. Unless a child is showing that they are having trouble breathing or other complications, treat this at home. If a child *is* having any trouble breathing or any unusual or worrying symptoms, call a doctor.

See the Colds and Flu section for more ideas on how to treat uncomplicated cases of RSV.

Pneumonia

While uncommon, pneumonia can be a complication of any respiratory infection in a child (or adult). It is an infection in the lungs and can make breathing difficult, cause cough and fever, and can take a few weeks to recover from. It is common to cough up mucus, and it may be green or rusty-colored. The child will probably be very tired or weak, and may experience diarrhea or vomiting[291].

Most cases of pneumonia are not dangerous and can be treated at home. Young babies or those with compromised immune systems may need more help – young babies who struggle to breathe should be seen by a doctor. A chest x-ray or a blood test can be used to diagnose it. In severe cases, that may require hospitalization, a chest x-ray can help to definitely confirm so that antibiotics are not offered unnecessarily[292]. Other doctors disagree and believe that chest x-rays may lead to more frequent diagnosis, since "white spots" (congestion) can show up for many reasons besides pneumonia[293]. A physical exam with listening to the chest may be enough.

Zinc supplementation may reduce the risk of pneumonia, if offered at the onset of cold or flu. It may also reduce inflammation and help the pneumonia heal[294]. Antibiotics are usually used with bacterial pneumonia, but may not be needed if it is not severe. Supportive care and home remedies can be used instead in many cases.

- **Bromelain** – This is an enzyme found in fresh pineapple and papaya. It can reduce the amount of mucus being produced and thin it for easier expulsion. (Try fresh pineapple juice and include the core, which is richest in bromelain.)

- **Juicing** -- Try adding carrot, beet, ginger, and parsley to the pineapple juice to help even more; especially since the patient probably does not want to eat. These are known to help detox the body.

- **Goldenseal** – This is a naturally antibiotic herb and can help fight pneumonia.

- **Probiotics** – Good bacteria, especially lactobacillus, has been shown to reduce respiratory infections in children[295].

- **Garlic** – This can be taken internally or made into a paste for the chest. It is anti-bacterial and anti-viral and can help the person overcome pneumonia faster. It may also be put on the feet for small babies who can't take it internally.

- **Ginger** – This is a warming remedy and it can help respiratory infections and reduce inflammation. Try it in a tea.

- **Fenugreek** – This helps the mucus to thin out as well as increasing perspiration to

---

291   http://www.webmd.com/lung/tc/pneumonia-topic-overview
292   http://journals.lww.com/pec-online/Abstract/2012/07000/Diagnosis_of_Childhood_Pneumonia__Clinical.9.aspx
293   http://www.rogerknapp.com/medical/pneumonia.htm
294   http://www.healthy.net/scr/Article.aspx?Id=3168
295   http://www.bmj.com/content/322/7298/1327

help detox the body and end the fever faster (but naturally). Take as a tea.

If pneumonia is not severe or is confirmed to be viral, try the remedies above. If the child is breathing shallowly or rapidly or struggling to breathe, or there are any other signs of complications, take the child to the doctor. Suction and oxygen as supportive care may be required. This is not too common in healthy older children.

Croup

This is common with colds in younger children. It is a severe, barking cough that sounds "seal-like" and usually occurs because of tiny breathing passages. It is most common in infants up through age 3, and it usually is worst at night. It typically lasts 1 – 3 days and may be accompanied by fever. It can be scary for the child, who may struggle to breathe or breathe in stridently after a coughing bout. Children who are truly having trouble breathing should be seen by a doctor. Otherwise, it can be treated at home. In addition to the suggestions in the Colds and Flu section, you may try:

- **Cool air** – Children with croup often benefit from breathing in cool air, which helps soothe inflamed breathing passages. Taking children outside in appropriate weather (usually at night) can help, or possibly sleeping with a window partially open.

- **Cool mist humidifier** – Using a cool mist humidifier can do a lot of what cool air can do, but can be used in any weather.

- **Eucalyptus oil** – This essential oil can help to clear breathing passages and make breathing easier. Use in a humidifier or place a drop on a child's pillow. Do not use directly on the child without diluting.

- **Sleep position** – Croup is usually worse at night, while lying down. Sleeping at an angle may help the child get more rest. Older children can simply use extra pillows. Younger babies may need to be held.

- **Mullein** – This herb soothes the respiratory tract and can help calm the coughing.

Constipation

Unfortunately, constipation is common among children (and adults). It is often caused by poor diet, one which is high in refined carbs and low in healthy fats. For most children, helping it is not too difficult. Children who have ongoing or severe problems or who are withholding feces due to constipation should be seen by a doctor.

Ideally, a child (and adult) should need to go two to three times a day, after every meal. They should need to go at least once per day. If a child is going infrequently, constipation may be suspected. Most doctors do not consider a person constipated unless the stool is passed with difficulty and is hard, suggesting a slow transit time in the intestines. Even sub-optimal elimination can be addressed by the measures below to improve health. Remember that feces are a waste product and should not stay in the body too long. Several days is too long.

- **Probiotics** – One of the best ways to promote digestive regularity is by adding probiotics to the diet. This includes probiotic foods like yogurt, kefir, kombucha, and fermented veggies, as well as probiotic supplements. Start slowly and increase the dose, because too much at once can cause diarrhea.

- **Coconut oil** – Eating this oil can help to increase the fat in the diet and may help ease constipation.
- **Eliminating 'binding' foods** – This includes bananas, potatoes, and other foods known to specifically alleviate diarrhea. Too much may cause constipation. The same goes for sugar and refined grains.
- **Water** – Sometimes, dehydration or drinking too little water can cause constipation, because all the water is pulled out to be used by the body. Drink more to see if this helps.
- **Vitamin C** – Enough of this can loosen the bowels.
- **Magnesium** – Epsom salts and other forms of magnesium are mild laxatives that can be used if needed.

These are the safest remedies. If anything strong is needed, please seek the advice of a medical professional. Laxatives can be habit-forming and may damage the child's body if used too often, and should not be used except under the direction of a medical professional.

As with anything, if you have a question about a remedy or your child's case, ask a professional.

A few children unfortunately suffer from some chronic conditions. These conditions may be managed in a number of different ways. Although all children who suffer from a chronic illness should be under a doctor's care, there are often holistic alternatives that may be combined with conventional therapies or, in some cases, may even take the place of conventional therapies. Always talk to a doctor or qualified health professional before changing or stopping a child's medication.

There are a number of other conditions that aren't included here. Chronic illness in and of itself could be an entire book! Some of the interventions mentioned here may be beneficial in other conditions as well. Seek the care and advice of an alternative doctor to learn which interventions may be beneficial in your child's case.

Asthma

This is a chronic lung condition that can cause "attacks" where a child's breathing becomes very difficult. Typically, steroid inhalers are used to help keep a child breathing well, and epinephrine is administered at the hospital in case of an attack. One small problems is that the inhalers that are used can cause "rebound" attacks. Children should have them to use in emergencies, but there are other remedies that may improve a child's lung function and reduce dependence on them.

- **Lobelia** – This herb can help reduce inflammation in lungs and improve breathing. Used as a tincture is easiest, and it should not be heated, as this destroys its beneficial properties.

- **Allergenic foods** – Some children have reduced asthma symptoms by avoiding foods that are triggers, especially gluten or dairy.

- **Avoid pollution** – Keep the home clean, get rid of pets if their dander is a trigger, use an air filter to reduce allergens. Do not smoke around children with asthma, as this can irritate lungs.

- **Coltsfoot** – This herb can reduce coughing, calm inflammation, and is good for bronchial passages. Make a tea from this herb and drink as needed, for any tightness or minor issues (not acute attacks).

- **Fenugreek** – This herb is also soothing to throats and bronchial passages and reduces mucus production, as well as soothing mucous membranes. It also tastes nice and may be easier for children to take.

- **Lemon balm** – This herb is anti-inflammatory and also anti-spasmodic, making it useful for lung conditions (also colds and flu) and can help to calm minor symptoms.

- **FCLO** – This supplement can raise vitamin D levels. Uncontrolled or severe asthma has been associated with low vitamin D levels[296] (which also increase the risk of developing asthma).

Autism

This is an incredibly complex neurological disorder that can cause a number of different

---

296   http://www.ncbi.nlm.nih.gov/pmc/articles/PMC2812815/

symptoms and can have a wide range of severity. I could write an entire book just about this. The current, official explanation is "we don't know." This is frustrating to many parents because there is very little support for autism therapies. Only behavioral therapies have been widely accepted (ABA, plus OT, PT, etc.). Biomedical interventions are written off as "possibly helpful; undetermined" through "useless and potentially detrimental," depending on which intervention it is and who you ask.

There is a movement right now to help children through dietary and other natural interventions. DAN doctors (Defeat Autism Now) are the primary practitioners in this area, although by no means the only ones. Seeking a DAN doctor may be a good idea if your child has autism and you are looking for alternative ideas. A DAN doctor can tailor a treatment program to your individual child. A chiropractor or other alternative health practitioner may also prove helpful, depending on your child's needs and the resources available in your community.

It is impossible to detail all of the potential interventions here, but there are a few common ones.

- **GF/CF Diet** – This stands for gluten-free/casein-free (dairy free). It removes all gluten-containing grains and all dairy from the diet. Many children, who may suffer from intolerances to these foods, have seen improvements from this diet.

- **GAPS** – Some children have more gut damage and a GF/CF diet alone isn't enough. The GAPS protocol calls for the removal of all grains, dairy, and focuses heavily on fat, meat stock, and probiotics in order to heal the gut and remove toxins. It was created by Dr. Natasha Campbell-McBride, who healed her son's autism with it. There are no official studies, but there are miraculous anecdotal stories.

- **Chelation** – Some children have mercury or other heavy metal toxicity. Chelation therapy is used to remove these heavy metals from the body to give the child a chance to heal.

- **Vitamin D** – There is some evidence that low vitamin D levels may play some role in autism. Supplementing with fish oils or cod liver oils to provide vitamin D as well as omega-3s (which may also play a role in autism) can help to relieve some symptoms.

ADHD

This is a common diagnosis now among children, sometimes as young as two years old. In many cases, the child may or may not actually have ADHD. Sometimes, a child is diagnosed because they don't "fit the mold" of a typical child – they have too much energy, they refuse to follow directions, they don't like to sit still or be quiet, and they don't seem to focus on activities that don't interest them. This may be developmental immaturity (since younger kids in every grade level are more likely to be labeled than older kids) or it may be that the child has a different learning style. An ADHD diagnosis may not be the right fit, and the stimulant medications used may not be the right answer – they can be dangerous.

For many children, symptoms can be improved by a number of more natural interventions.

- **Developmental maturity** – Some children need more time to mature than others.

It is not necessarily a sign of a problem, especially if the child is under 6 or 7 years old.

- **Unique learning style** – Some children benefit from a more physical, hands-on learning experience and don't do well with needing to sit still and listen. If possible, look for an alternative schooling situation. This is especially helpful if your child does not appear to display any symptoms at home/on the weekends but struggles during school hours.

- **Feingold diet** – This diet removes artificial flavors and colors and other food additives, as well as salicylates from the diet, with the idea that these particular foods trigger symptoms in children.

- **Sugar** – Although supposedly disproven that sugar causes hyperactivity in children, it can spike blood sugar and lead to a pattern of "highs" and "crashes" and this sort of imbalance may lead to symptoms.

- **Vitamin D** – Some evidence shows that vitamin D may help children to focus better. Omega-3s, found in cod liver oil, may also help some children.

Diabetes

More children have diabetes today than ever before. More of them are also ending up with type II diabetes, which used to be called "adult onset." Vitamin D deficiency, which is rampant, has been linked to both type I and type II, and it increases the chances of getting diabetes[297]. The primary way to prevent diabetes is to make sure the child isn't deficient in vitamin D, and also to focus on a healthy diet – one that doesn't restrict (healthy) fat, but does restrict sugar and refined carbs. There are ways to help diabetes if a child has been diagnosed. Talk to your child's doctor before adjusting his/her diet or adding in herbs.

- **Vitamin D** – Since deficiency is linked to poor management/difficulty in controlling diabetes, supplementing to achieve optimal levels is important.

- **No refined sugar/grains** – Children should consume whole grains and minimal amounts of natural sugars only, to prevent blood sugar spikes.

- **Fenugreek** – Used as a tea, it helps to stabilize blood sugar.

- **Healthy fat** – Include coconut oil, butter, and other saturated and monounsaturated fats, which help the child's body anyway and may also help balance blood sugar and reduce sugar cravings.

- **Probiotics** – Friendly bacteria is always beneficial, and it may help to balance the gut and reduce symptoms.

Lyme Disease

Lately, there has been concern over Lyme disease. It is caused by deer tick bites and can cause serious problems for months or years, especially since it is rarely detected or diagnosed very easily. The standard treatment right now is at least a month of antibiotics, and this may or may not be effective. People struggle with ongoing joint pain, fatigue, fever, muscle aches, headaches, sometimes a "bullseye" rash, and other

---

297   http://www.ncbi.nlm.nih.gov/pubmed/15971062

serious issues because of Lyme. There are some natural remedies that may help.

- **Goldenseal** – This herb is a natural antibiotic and a traditional treatment for Lyme disease and other conditions. It is most effective when used as close to the onset of symptoms as possible. It also reduces inflammation in the body, which is common with Lyme.
- **Vitamin C** – This may help your body boost its defenses, which can help fight off Lyme disease. High doses may be used at least initially.
- **Coconut oil** – This is anti-viral and contains an important medium-chain fatty acid, lauric acid. This acid in particular may help to fight Lyme disease. There is also a supplement called "monolaurin" which is basically concentrated lauric acid.
- **Cat's Claw** – This herb may target tick-borne illness and help to eliminate Lyme disease.
- **Vitamin D** – A deficiency lowers the immune system, making recovery more difficult. Supplementing may help.
- **Vitamin B complex** – Especially B12, but also others. Deficiencies in B vitamins are common with Lyme, and some research suggests that Lyme may exacerbate B vitamin deficiency.

If possible, seek the help of a qualified alternative practitioner to help you address your personal issues. You may require other treatments, depending on the severity of symptoms and the length of time symptoms have been going on. Natural treatment is possible!

WHEN TO CALL THE DOCTOR

If you've learned anything while reading this book, it's that there's a time and a place when the doctor should be called. Doctors don't need to be consulted for every sniffle and slight fever, but there are definitely times when they are needed. Doctors, after all, specialize in sick care, and when a child is very ill and home remedies aren't working quickly, then a doctor is the best person to turn to.

How do you know if it's serious enough to call a doctor, though?

First of all, if in doubt – always call. Ask for a consultation over the phone with the doctor or a nurse in his/her office and explain your child's symptoms. Ask for advice on dealing with them or if an appointment is warranted. This avoids an automatic appointment (and the co-pays and time associated with it), but gives you the peace of mind that your child's doctor is aware of the situation, in case anything more serious develops. If you do call, always ask "What symptoms should I be looking for to indicate that this is serious? If I see them, should I call you back for an appointment or take the child to urgent care or the emergency room?" Know how your doctor wants the situation handled if something does go wrong.

Signs You Need to Call the Doctor

Remember that calling doesn't mean that you have to follow the doctor's advice 100%. But it can give you the peace of mind to know if what your child is experiencing is really a problem or not, and give you an idea on how to treat it. If you are concerned about the advice your doctor may give you (i.e. that it won't be "naturally inclined") you may look for an alternative doctor whose practice is more in line with your beliefs.

- **Fever in a young baby** – Any fever in a baby under three months warrants a call to a doctor, especially if the baby has other symptoms. Small babies can become very ill very rapidly because of their underdeveloped immune systems. Most say if the baby's temperature reaches 100.4 to call.

- **Persistent vomiting or diarrhea** – If it lasts more than 6 to 12 hours OR if the child is beginning to show any signs of dehydration, a call is warranted, and IV fluids may be needed.

- **Dehydration** – If the child's skin is "pinchable" (pinch it and it doesn't immediately 'snap' back but moves slowly), the child's mouth is dry, eyes look sunken, etc. try to rehydrate the child. If nothing changes within 30 minutes, call. If the baby is a young infant, call immediately.

- **Lethargy** – A child who is tired/wants to rest is fine; a child who seems unable to get up or unusually weak is not. Call if the child's weakness is worrying.

- **High-pitched screaming** – This can be a sign of encephalitis and should be taken seriously. Especially if it is accompanied by a high fever, call, and the child may need to be seen immediately.

- **Unresponsive** – A child who does not focus on you when you call (eyes not looking), does not answer you, otherwise does not respond, may need to be seen immediately. Call.

- **Seizures** – Call and ask what to do. A doctor may not want to see a child if they suspect it is a febrile seizure, but any other form of seizure or repeated seizures warrants a visit to a doctor.
- **Bleeding** – Any serious bleeding, that is. A paper cut is obviously fine, but bleeding that is not stopping easily with pressure, or which is unexplained (i.e. no injury) warrants a call.
- **Serious injuries** – If your child sustains any sort of injury, either call the doctor or take the child to the emergency room, depending on the nature of the injury. (Broken bones obviously require a trip to the emergency room, as does serious bleeding.)
- **Unexplained/frequent bruising** – Call someone. As this may be a sign of cancer, anemia, or any number of other serious illnesses, the child should probably be seen. Be aware that if the worst were to happen and the child were diagnosed with cancer by a mainstream doctor, they would be legally required to undergo chemo or whatever the "standard protocol" is for that type of cancer. If this is something you are opposed to, seek care from an alternative doctor if possible. Parents who do not cooperate with the "standard of care" in serious cases like cancer can and have had children's services called.
- **Frequent fevers** – Fevers which occur on a regular basis may also be a sign of something more serious, and the child should be seen.
- **Head injury** – If a child has a head injury, especially if they seem unusually tired or lethargic after, call. (A minor bump on the head followed by normal behavior is probably fine.)
- **Acting "not right"** – If something in your mother instincts tells you "this just isn't right," call. It is better to be safe than sorry.

This is not an exhaustive list of when to call the doctor, but it covers most of the "big" ones. Always remember to call if you are worried.

Ideally, develop a relationship with a doctor that you trust, and seek his/her counsel when treating an ill child. Some parents choose a naturopath or chiropractor for this purpose. See the section on alternative doctors.

ALTERNATIVE DOCTORS

In addition to mainstream pediatricians, there are several alternative doctors out there. These alternative doctors may be a better fit for families who prefer to avoid medication or have a "holistic" bent – even those who prefer to *sometimes* avoid medication may like having a naturally-minded doctor. Having a doctor that you can trust can be extremely beneficial on the occasions when a child has a serious enough problem that home care isn't enough. Knowing that the doctor is going to thoroughly investigate the child's symptoms and not be too quick to recommend drugs is even better.

There are several types of alternative doctors out there that warrant mentioning.

Holistic Pediatrician

There are board-certified pediatricians out there who choose to practice more holistically. They are "normal" pediatricians who hold an MD or DO and who have gone through a residency. They can prescribe drugs, but they tend not to do so too quickly. These pediatricians tend to take longer to examine children during appointments and take on fewer patients. They often recommend supplements and home treatments instead of jumping to medication, although they will prescribe it when they feel it is warranted. These pediatricians are excellent to have but often difficult to find.

Family Doctors

While not necessarily holistic (you'll have to interview them), family doctors do tend to take a more relaxed approach to health than pediatricians, as a generalization. For those who feel they need a "mainstream" doctor and who cannot find a holistic pediatrician, a family doctor may be a good solution. Family doctors treat people of all ages rather than specializing in children and so may be more approachable about various issues.

Naturopath

This is not a regulated term, per se. In some states, naturopaths are recognized and licensed; in others they are not. A naturopath is anyone who practices some form of holistic medicine. This person may have been through a rigorous academic program of some kind, or may have been through a short correspondence school. (In states where this isn't recognized, almost anyone can claim to be a naturopath.) Ask to see the person's credentials. Naturopaths in general look for dietary interventions first, and also recommend supplements, herbs, and other natural cures.

Homeopath

A homeopath has been to a two to four year school that teaches classical homeopathy. Homeopathy uses very dilute substances that have been "succussed" (shaken) to increase potency. These substances are used in tiny amounts with the theory that "like cures like." (Basically, they boost the body's immune reaction slightly, helping it to heal faster.) Remedies are based on the person's symptoms, personality, and other individual factors, not a disease or condition name. A classical homeopath will get to know a patient thoroughly and will recommend a single remedy that best fits that person's situation. There are some different schools of thought on homeopathy and how to select and give remedies, so remember that when choosing a homeopath. Conventional doctors believe homeopathy does not work but many others believe differently[298].

Chiropractic

A chiropractor is a doctor who specializes in external manipulation of the spine. Nerves are connected to the spine and the messages to various parts of the body flow from the brain, down the spine, to the proper nerves. A spine which is misaligned (out of position) can affect the way the messages flow down the nerves and interrupt them. Depending on the issue, there can be pain involved. Chiropractic is helpful to maintain optimal health as a preventative measure, and can also help with pain, ear infections (by re-aligning the ears so they drain), and a number of other issues.

Nutritional Response Testing

This has to do with muscle testing, a method of determining the body's sensitivities to certain substances. The substance is placed against the body and if the arm, when pushed on, goes weak, the body is sensitive. The body diverts blood and energy from the arm to the vital organs to combat the "threat" of the substance. There are various other ways to do this (checking different organs, testing for the presence of infection, dealing with food allergies). These doctors usually recommend dietary changes and supplements to help heal the body, and some practice NAET[299].

Other

There are other alternative doctors as well – health coaches, Reiki, Chinese medicine, acupuncture, and so on. These are used less commonly and mostly by adults, which is why this book does not discuss them in-depth. There may be a time and place to seek these other alternative practices, especially with older children. Ask for referrals, if needed, from other alternative doctors in your area.

Remember that when choosing an alternative doctor in any area, there are good ones and bad ones, as in any other profession. An entire field should not be written off because of one bad practitioner. If the first one that you find is not a good fit for your family, keep looking. All doctors practice a bit differently, no matter what their field, and should be evaluated based on their individual education, personality, and general merit.

Our personal choice is a chiropractor, whom our children see one or two times a month for regular "check ups." They see a holistic pediatrician annually. We consult with a Nutritional Response Testing doctor every now and then if allergy issues crop up (my husband sees this doctor regularly, but the kids don't). These are our choices, based on who is available in our area and what we feel works for our family. Everyone will be different.

---

298   http://www.homeorizon.com/homeopathic-articles/homeopathic-researches/efficacy-of-homoe-opathy
299   http://www.naet.com/

HERB GUIDE

A lot of parents who are new to alternative medicine are very uncertain about herbs. Which are safe? Which are beneficial? What are they for?

While I am not a trained herbalist and there are literally thousands of herbs out there, this is a brief rundown of some basics herbs that may be used in children's alternative medicine. For additional information, please check with a master herbalist or other alternative health practitioner. If your child has special medical conditions or medical needs, please do not assume any herb is safe without consulting an expert.

Alfalfa

This is a green herb that is nourishing and adaptogenic in nature. It is high in vitamin K especially and can be used to increase vitamin K stores if needed. It also contains many other vitamins and minerals and can be safely prepared as a general herbal tea for children.

Aloe Vera

This is a cactus that contains a soothing liquid that can be applied to burned skin or otherwise irritated skin. It can also be drunk in small quantities to aid digestive health. Small children should not use it internally and older children should start with only a teaspoon or two per day.

Arnica

This herb should not be used orally. It can help soothe sore muscles and general pain when used as a salve or cream. The only exception to the oral use is in homeopathic form, but *never* use home preparations from the whole herb orally.

Bee Pollen

This is the pollen from a beehive. It's best if it is local and it can help allergies as well as boosting immunity. Start with only 1 – 2 granules per day in children over a year old and work up to a teaspoon or so. Older children and adults can take a tablespoon after building up.

Calendula

This is an herb that is nourishing and healing for the skin. It is the yellow calendula flowers. It is good when added to skin creams (infused in the oils) or if a salve is made from it. It can be used for eczema and diaper rash.

Catnip

This herb is a mild sedative and is good for helping children relax. It can help hyper children calm down and can induce sleep as well. It is one of the safest sedatives because it is so mild and can be used in babies. Paired with cloves, it is a big help with teething.

Chamomile

This herb is also a mild sedative and is known for helping children calm down and prepare for sleep. It can safely be used in a tea form for nearly any age. It can also soothe digestive distress in some cases.

Cloves

This herb – whole cloves – is good for oral pain. Any sort of jaw tension, infections or, most commonly, teething. Paired with catnip and made into a tea, it can soothe sore gums and help teething babies rest more easily.

Comfrey

This herb should not be used internally. It is good for soothing and healing skin, and may be used in skin creams, hair rinses, salves, and more.

Devil's Claw

This herb is an anti-inflammatory herb which may be beneficial in pain relief. It tends to be safe and has not shown to be toxic even in large doses. It can be used topically or in a tincture.

Echinacea

This herb is known to help boost immunity during colds and flu and to help the person recover faster. It should be used only during illness and for no longer than two weeks at a time. Longer uses may render the herb ineffective or even toxic. It can be prepared as a tea for younger children and may be taken in capsules by older children, if desired.

Fennel

This herb is known to increase milk supply in lactating women, but it also has anti-nausea properties. It can be crushed and used as a tea for stomachaches and colic in babies. Paired with ginger, it makes "gripe water," a popular colic and gas remedy.

Fenugreek

This herb is most popularly known to increase milk supply in lactating women, but it has many other uses. In children, the most common use is for colds and sore throats. It can relieve the discomfort from a sore throat as well as helping to eliminate mucus from the body more effectively, easing cold or pneumonia symptoms. It can be prepared as a tea or included in a homemade cold syrup.

Garlic

This is one of the most common herbs because it is very safe (used in cooking, and not really possible to overdose). It is antibacterial, antiviral, and antifungal. It can be consumed orally to help combat infections. It can be mixed with coconut oil and rubbed onto the feet to combat infections as well, especially in young children. It can be mixed with a liquid oil and dropped into the ears to help ear infections. Although usually too strong, it could also help fungal infections on the skin if mixed with a carrier oil.

Ginger

This is a very popular and very safe herb. It can even be used in newborns. Ginger can help sore throats, colds, coughs, ease congestion, soothe digestive upset, boost overall liver function, reduce inflammation and relieve pain, and more. In small children it is most often used for colic or gas. It can be made into a tea or tincture.

Goldenseal

This is a very expensive herb that can be used topically to heal skin inflammation and rashes. It is commonly used on diaper rash, and can be used by itself as a powder or added to salves or creams. Do not use internally unless directed by an herbalist.

Lemon balm

This is an herb in the mint family which is very safe. It has been said to help colds, coughs, and digestive upset. It can be made into a safe herbal tea for children and is even a good substitute for "lemonade" in the summer, when paired with a bit of stevia or raw honey.

Mullein

This herb is extremely versatile and also safe for children. It can be used to address viral infections, respiratory infections, diarrhea, migraines, and many other conditions. It is a good addition to the medicine cabinet because it has so many uses.

Nettles

This is an herb commonly known as "stinging nettle." It is a rich source of vitamins and minerals and may be beneficial for seasonal allergies. It can be prepared as a general herbal tea.

Oatstraw

This is an herb related to oats (it's part of the oat plant). It is rich in vitamins and minerals and is beneficial to the skin. A strong tea of oatstraw can be added to a bath to relieve itching in case of infection, eczema, or otherwise. It can also be consumed as a tea.

Passion Flower

This is a stronger sedative and induces relaxation and sleep. Chamomile or catnip are preferable, but passion flower may be an option for children who do not respond to these or who have a serious need for sleep and rest.

Peppermint

This is a safe herb that is cooling and soothing for skin as well as anti-nausea. It can be consumed as a tea or used in salves. Be careful when adding it to a bath as it can be very strong and cooling and may be uncomfortable. The tea form can be consumed hot or cold simply for enjoyment.

Red Clover

This herb is the blossoms of red clover and can be found growing wildly in many areas in the late spring and early summer months. It has estrogenic properties and generally should not be used for children, although some women may benefit from it.

Red Raspberry Leaf

This herb is commonly used in pregnant women because it relaxes the smooth muscles. It is okay for children to have on occasion – for example, if mom is drinking it and they want some. It is rich in vitamins and minerals as well.

Skullcap

This is another mild sedative and may be useful in hyperactive children or those who have difficulty focusing. It can be used in a teething tea in place of catnip.

Spearmint

This is an herb in the mint family which is a bit milder than peppermint. It can be used for tea and is high in B vitamins (including folate) as well as other vitamins and minerals. It may be beneficial in combating nausea. It can be enjoyed as a tea as desired.

Valerian

This is a much stronger sedative for those who really struggling with sleep. It may be habit-forming and should be a last resort. It also is very strong-smelling and most people don't like it.

EXERCISE AND MOTION

There's a big focus right now on getting kids to exercise more. A lack of exercise is being blamed for the obesity crisis that we face. While exercise does play a role there, diet is a much more pressing concern. Still, it's true that kids are getting less and less time outdoors and in motion – and they need this time for proper development. More and more kids are also considered a "problem" if they have a lot of energy, and are being drugged with Ritalin and Adderall instead of being allowed to have an appropriate physical outlet. Physical activity is extremely important.

The average healthy child has trouble sitting still and needs to be in frequent motion. They could use 2 – 4 hours per day of some sort of physical activity – running, jumping, climbing, dancing, and so on. Healthy children spend almost all their time moving, eating, or sleeping – and sometimes more than one at once! They have a strong need to fuel their bodies and then burn off the energy and this need shouldn't be thwarted.

Children should, if possible, have an appropriate outdoor play space. They should be encouraged to run, climb, ride bikes, and otherwise participate in physical games, both alone and in collaboration with others.

Indoors, children should have physical options as well. A small indoor climbing structure is a good idea, or an open area in which they can run. Children will often find something to climb on or be physical with if they are not provided with appropriate alternatives! A dedicated play area with some sort of "physical" options is a good idea. Older children (8 or so) can use small hand weights, jump ropes, or mini-trampolines.

Some children enjoy organized physical activity – sports teams, gymnastics or dance classes, swimming lessons, and so on. Children who are interested in these should be encouraged to participate if possible.

Physical activity is a real need; not merely a desire. Children shouldn't be asked to "sit down and be quiet" too often. Children who do not seem to desire physical activity in some form very often should be checked out – most young children have boundless energy, and they should.

For older children, fitness should be encouraged and modeled by parents. Encourage children to play backyard games, jump on trampolines (safely!), or take on whatever exercise they prefer. Taking walks as a family is a great way to get everyone moving. It's good to focus on health as the reason for exercise, especially with pre-teens and teens – it should not be about weight or body image. We exercise so we feel good, not because we hate our bodies. For parents who have always struggled with body image and feelings of inadequacy from being overweight, this may be difficult – but it's good to shift focus!

Exercise doesn't have to be complicated. It should fit the family's lifestyle and simply be a part of what you "do." This way children will grow up with a healthy attitude towards exercise and fitness.

SECTION 3: ENVIRONMENT

DO YOU NEED ORGANIC BEDS AND BEDDING?

When a baby is coming – or when a baby has become a toddler and is ready to move into his own "big kid bed" – there comes the question, is it worth it to spend the money on an organic bed and bedding?

The Case for Organic

Some parents come down staunchly on the side that yes, this is necessary. There are several reasons why this is.

Babies and kids spend a *lot* of time sleeping. A newborn may sleep up to 18 hours out of every 24, and toddlers and older children may sleep 11 – 14 hours out of every 24. That's 50 – 75% of their time, spent in contact with that mattress and bedding!

This may not be a problem, except that regular mattresses contain potentially toxic flame retardants. There is a group of chemicals called PDBEs that are used in mattresses, car seats, and other furniture in order to slow down flames, should these items catch fire (also children's pajamas). These chemicals have been used for over 30 years now. The problem is, they've been associated with problems with human health.

These chemicals are somewhat similar to BPA and they have potential estrogenic effects[300]. It has also been linked to low birth weight[301] when mothers have the chemicals concentrated in their bodies (which occurs when they sleep on the mattresses coated with them). There is also some evidence linking them to liver toxicity, thyroid damage, developmental changes, and neurotoxicity[302].

PDBEs are added to fabric and can (and do) off-gas into the environment, and are therefore present in most homes. They enter the body when we breathe them in or when our skin is in contact with the clothes or furniture, and they don't tend to be excreted easily at all, which means they can build up in the body over time[303]. Unfortunately, despite mounting evidence of harm, this information is being suppressed by the chemical industry, who says there is "no proven danger."

Crib mattresses may also contain arsenic and formaldehyde, which are also toxic, especially to young children with developing brains and bodies.

Organic mattresses, bedding, and clothing do not contain these chemicals, which is many parents' main reason for choosing them. Some mattresses also claim to be better support for the body, healthier for posture, and this may factor into some parents' choice as well.

Organic mattresses are still flame-retardant, but they achieve this using natural wool, not chemicals. The wool is also resistant to mold, dust mites, and mildew – making it easier to clean and better for those with allergies. Other materials used include natural rubber and natural latex.

When it comes to organic bedding, there are some different issues. Cotton is one of

300   http://www.ncbi.nlm.nih.gov/pmc/articles/PMC1240281/
301   http://www.ncbi.nlm.nih.gov/pubmed/21878423
302   http://www.ncbi.nlm.nih.gov/pmc/articles/PMC1367864/
303   http://www.naturepedic.com/education/quotes.php

the most heavily-sprayed crops out there. There may be residue left in the cotton after processing (depends on who you ask), and purchasing "normal" sheets certainly contributes to the growing of conventional cotton.

The Case Against Organic

The major case against organic is that it's expensive. Very expensive. A "normal" crib mattress may cost $50 - $200, depending on quality. Organic crib mattresses start around $300 and can be up to $500, occasionally more.

Beds for older children start around $1000 (compared to $xxx for standard mattresses), and depending on quality, materials, and size, can be up to $4000. For many parents, especially those with several children, this is cost-prohibitive. As much as parents would like to buy "the best of everything," they simply cannot afford to spend that much money on each child's bed – not to mention their own.

There are ways to compromise.

If only one mattress can be purchased organically, make it the crib mattress. It's the cheapest of the options, and babies spend a lot more time sleeping than older children do – plus, their bodies are less developed and more fragile. $400 for an organic crib mattress may be doable, even if $1000 for a twin-sized mattress isn't. Plus, the crib mattress can be reused on multiple babies, making it even more cost-effective (vs. a twin bed that the child will likely sleep in until grown, necessitating a separate purchase for each).

That's still a lot for families to pay and may not be feasible in all cases. Another compromise is to buy a wool-based organic mattress cover, which run between $20 and $50 each. This is much more affordable and at least for new babies, could even be added to a baby registry. This pad protects the mattress from any diaper leaks, accidents, or spills, and it also helps the off-gassing issue.

Organic crib sheets aren't much more expensive than "regular" ones. A typical crib sheet cost $10 - $30, depending on brand, materials, etc. An organic crib sheet may cost $15 - $30 – so, this is fairly affordable.

As for organic sheets for larger beds, they vary from $40 - $100 (or so). They can be obtained for about the same price as a conventional, high-quality sheet set. It would be worth it, if possible, to get two good sheet sets for each bed – nice quality, and no extra clutter!

If possible, try to do what you can to minimize the toxins in the sleep environment. When mattresses are new, keep windows open for awhile (if it's not too cold) to let them air out. Consider vacuuming them or using an air filter. Cover them with a wool mattress cover or topper. Use the best sheets you can afford. High quality lasts longer anyway!

Know what the situation is, but don't worry too much if you can't choose "best." There are limited resources, limited money, and we all do what we can.

At this time we don't have any organic beds or bedding. We have chosen to keep and re-used older mattresses (from family members) which no longer off-gas very much. We are considering adding the wool mattress pads and hope to purchase organic mattresses if we can afford to in the future.

CHOOSING SAFE CLOTHING

As mentioned in the previous section, there are two major issues with clothing: the fact that many are made from conventional cotton (a heavily-sprayed crop) and that pajamas are coated in flame retardants. This is required for any clothing that is intended to be used as sleep wear.

Many parents want their children to have safe clothing. Since children grow rapidly, spending hundreds to thousands of dollars on a wardrobe their child will wear for only a year (or less) is hardly feasible. Organic outfits can run from $5 per item on up to $20 or more. Some parents may be able to afford this or may choose to prioritize it.

Others may get involved in a "clothing swap" where several friends or family members pass clothing from one family to another as they are outgrown so that everyone can benefit from high-quality clothing without having to pay the price tag alone.

If organic clothing – or at least an entire wardrobe of organic clothing – is out of the question, there are still ways to obtain safer clothing items.

Pajamas

These are probably one of the biggest concerns, since they contain the flame retardants (see the section on Organic Beds and Bedding for more on those). All clothing that is intended for use as sleep wear and which is not organic must contains these chemicals. One solution is to buy all organic pajamas. These can run $15 - $35 *per pair*, and probably more – not so feasible for most families.

Another solution is to buy used pajamas from a thrift store. They have likely been washed many times and the chemicals have been mostly washed out of them. Wash them at home in hot water with a natural detergent and allow them to dry in the sun, if possible. These should be fairly safe for most, and also extremely frugal.

A third solution is to buy clothes that are not intended for sleepwear. Our children largely wear plain t-shirts (used or organic undershirts aren't too expensive and we pass them down through all the kids as they're gender neutral and intended just for bed time) and sweatpants or used pajama pants for bed. They prefer this to one-piece or footie-style pajamas in most cases, and sweatpants can be subtracted in the summer (underwear or diaper + t-shirt) and a sweatshirt can be added in the winter so they work year around.

Other Clothing

Buying used or swapping with a friend and washing in natural detergent is going to be the most economical solution for most families. Check thrift stores, garage sales, consignment sales, and so on. Kids don't need a fancy or extensive wardrobe, and choosing to "keep it simple" with 5 – 7 of each major item is usually enough. (That is – pants, shirts, pairs of socks, underwear.) Specialty items, like holiday clothes, can often be swapped or purchased second-hand in very good condition for a low price, since these items are usually not worn very much.

Shoes

These are one thing worth buying new – at least one good pair of sneakers, ones they'll wear everyday. Shoes affect a child's physical development and should fit the child properly. Young children (not yet walking or early walkers) should not wear shoes or should choose flexible shoes. Barefoot is one of the safest and most important ways to walk[304]. Children should be encouraged to wear minimal footwear whenever possible, and to wear footwear that fits well when it is really required to have something on.

Special shoes that are worn infrequently (dress shoes, boots, etc.) can be purchased used or shared among family/friends as they don't affect a child's foot as much due to rare use. Children should not wear high heels (even when older) if at all possible because this is very bad for the feet, legs, and back. They can even cause permanent damage to the legs and knees[305].

Washing Clothes

Many parents want to know about safe detergents. This is the cleaning product that will come into contact with your child the most. There are detergent residues that stay in the clothing and which can absorb into your child's skin. Most detergents are harsh and are made from petroleum. Those scented detergents have even been shown to cause cancer[306].

Instead of choosing a typical detergent, look for something more natural. There are several different companies and products on the market now. There are also several recipes for homemade options.

The safest that I know of, and the one with which I am most familiar, is soap nuts. These are small, brown "nuts" that grow on soap berry trees. They are coated in a natural saponin. These soap nuts are tossed into a small muslin bag, which is added to the washing machine. They can be reused a few times to wash additional loads of clothing, and can be composted when they are spent. (They will be grayish and mushy and no longer feeling slippery.) They literally grow on trees and aren't processed at all, and they leave no residue in clothing.

These soap nuts have no scent, and can safely be used on cloth diapers as well. I have personally used them for almost five years on all my laundry and have preferred them. They have worked especially well for cloth diapers. While other natural detergents led to stinky diapers and a need to strip after awhile, soap nuts didn't. They are also quite frugal, available at Mountain Rose Herbs for $6/lb[307]. (This will last the average family 3 – 6 months.)

White vinegar is an effective laundry softener, if one is needed. Simply add it to the usual "softener dispenser" on the washer.

With safer, chemical-free laundry products, many people notice that dry skin and eczema lessen or disappear. Young, vulnerable children with thinner skin are also exposed to fewer toxic chemicals. Plus, the natural options are very easy to use. If the ones above don't work for you, try some of the popular brands until you find one that does: Seventh Generation, Mrs. Meyer's, Rockin' Green, and so on.

---

304   http://www.ncbi.nlm.nih.gov/pubmed/17353125
305   http://news.discovery.com/human/high-heels-legs-health.html
306   http://www.cbsnews.com/8301-504763_162-20097302-10391704.html
307   http://www.mountainroseherbs.com/bulkherb/s.php#h_s_so

Furniture is an easy area to overlook. We often already have some furniture that we can reuse, or we simply choose a set based on how nice it looks and how long it will last. However, there are several concerns relating to furniture.

Bedroom Furniture

This includes a crib, changing table, rocking chair or glider, and a dresser. There are several potential safety concerns with these.

First, all furniture should be in good condition. It should not have any sharp edges or broken pieces that a child could get hurt on. Cribs should be newer than 15 years old so they comply with current safety standards, and if you are buying second-hand, check to make sure that the crib hasn't been recalled. Cribs with cut-outs on the sides or where the bars are further apart than 2 3/8" do not meet current safety standards. Drop-side cribs are also no longer recommended[308] because they may have small metal parts on which a child's clothing could get caught, leading the child to strangle.

Changing tables and dressers should be heavy enough that a child could pull to stand on them, pull all the drawers out and shake them without being able to knock them over. If they are not this sturdy, they should be bolted to the wall to prevent falling.

If stained, the furniture should sit outside for several days after. Exposure to the fumes is toxic[309]. There are non-toxic stains to choose from instead, and this is a good idea especially for cribs, which children may chew on while teething.

Cribs should have mattresses that fit firmly and tightly in the space. Most sources advise against using crib bumpers anymore, because their use has been associated with strangulation or suffocation, especially in younger babies[310]. If they are used, they must have very short ties and must be tied firmly to the crib in all locations. (We do choose to use them, but only with older babies for whom suffocation is not much of an issue, and they are always tied tightly.)

Rocking chairs and gliders should have pads that tie onto the chair, if they have any. They should be placed in a location that a child can't crawl underneath them or get hurt on their moving parts. Do not let a child play unattended in a room with a glider once they are mobile.

High Chairs and Strollers

Most parents use these two items to help their children eat and get around. If you buy them secondhand, check to see if they were recalled for any reason. Use the safety straps on both to keep the child in place – many children learn to stand and can tip themselves out.

There are "high chairs" that are really booster seats with trays on them which strap onto chairs, which are space-savers (as they don't require a separate item) and can go from when babies can sit, around 6 months, on up to 3 – 4 years, when they outgrow a booster seat. Most of these can also be folded and taken along to restaurants or friends'

---

308   http://www.cbc.ca/news/health/story/2011/02/17/crib-injuries.html
309   http://www.nlm.nih.gov/medlineplus/ency/article/002825.htm
310   http://www.sciencedaily.com/releases/2007/09/070918165353.htm

houses, so they function well in many capacities. They are also usually very affordable.

Many parents choose to wear their babies in slings or wrap carriers of some type in addition to or instead of using a stroller. This is an excellent way to carry a baby and parents interested in baby wearing should look into it further and choose a high-quality carrier. Our preference was a Moby-style wrap carrier until around 6 months (or about 15 lbs., for our babies) and a Mei Tai-style carrier after that. Be wary of the Baby Bjorn and other popular carriers; these can be hard on the baby's hips because of the way it holds them. A more traditional carrier is safer.

Car Seats

This is one of the *biggest* safety issues with young children. Car accidents are the leading cause of death in children 1 to 12 years of age. Most parents do not use car seats appropriately, and this sharply increases the risk of injury or death if the child is in a car accident[311].

The absolute minimums (laws) are these:

- Children under 1 year AND 20 lbs. must be rear-facing
- Children up to 4 years AND 40 lbs. should be in forward-facing carseat with a 5-point harness
- Children should be in a booster until they are 8 years AND 80 lbs.

These standards are higher than when many parents were young – quite a bit, in some cases. Many of us were completely out of car seats by the time we were 3 – 4 years old. Current safety shows that this practice is *not* safe. It is never okay to reason "we all lived through it, and my kid will too." It is extremely important to follow the laws, which are only *minimum* safety standards.

The new safety standards (ideal) are these:

- Children should ride rear-facing until at least 2 years AND 30 lbs., or until the limits of the seat (many convertible seats now go up to 40 – 45 lbs. rear-facing)
- Children should be in a 5-pt. harness until they outgrow the seat (many seats go from 55 – 100 lbs.)
- Children should remain in a booster until they hit 80 lbs. or 4'9" tall

Many parents really balk at this. "But she won't have any leg room, she might break a leg!" or "Her friends will make fun of her!" or even "I'm barely 4'9" now, I wouldn't have been out of a car seat until I was a teen!"

This is about safety. This is about your child's life. If an accident occurs, there are no do-overs. There is no time to re-think and make your child safer in that moment. The only way to try to prevent a tragedy is by choosing to strap your child into an appropriate car seat, and use it properly, *every* time you are in the car. What your child's friends think does not matter (not to mention most of them are going to be in a car seat a lot longer, too).

There's no evidence that children – who are very flexible – are at risk of a broken leg while rear-facing. Even if they do, they are *far* less likely to break their necks. It is usually easy to fix a broken leg...it is nearly impossible to fix a broken neck.

---

311   http://www.nhtsa.gov/Safety/CPS

As for "My child is too large!" there are now car seats on the market to accommodate this. It's not about how large the child is, it is about their physical development. A 30-lb. 18-month-old and a 30-lb. 5-year-old are developmentally *very* different. The 5-year-old may be perfectly safe in a standard forward-facing car seat, while an 18-month-old wouldn't be. A young child's spine is so fragile that they can suffer from something called "internal decapitation," where their spinal cord separates from their brain, killing them. Watch this video[312] to see the difference in how a car crash affects a child in each position. It is about 500% safer to be rear-facing.

We personally chose to turn our children around when they reached 3 years old and 30 lbs. Yes, they were quite tall and no, their legs didn't fit. They crossed them or stuck them around the sides of the seat. At this point they were close to the max. rear-facing weight limit and they were also physically developed enough that we felt they would be safe enough if anything happened. Our 5-year-old is still in a normal forward-facing car seat and will be for another year or two, before moving to a booster.

Proper car seat use is also important. The right car seat won't do anything if it isn't installed and used correctly. Most parents don't use their seats correctly, which places children at an increased risk of injury.

Important things to know:

- The car seat must be tightly installed. It should not move more than 1" in either direction at the base. (Put your weight on it as you are pulling it tight with the seatbelt or the LATCH system to make sure it is really, truly tight.)
- Infant seats must be firmly clicked into the base.
- Use the correct belt path – one is labeled "rear facing" and one is labeled "forward facing."
- Make sure the car seat is at an appropriate angle, between 30 and 45 degrees. Most carseats have guides on them to show you how.
- Put the straps on the child tightly. If you can slip more than one finger beneath them, they are not tight enough.
- Do *not* put a child in a thick/puffy winter jacket in a carseat. These compress in an accident, making the straps loose, and the child could fly out. Use layers, a thin fleece jacket, or put a blanket on the child over the straps.
- Do not add any "after market" product to the seat. No seat cushions, no bundle wraps, nothing that goes under the straps. These can make the seat unsafe and they void your warranty.
- The chest clip goes high across the chest, *never* across the belly. In an accident it could press into a child's belly and bruise their internal organs...or worse.
- Make sure the straps are straight, never twisted.
- Insist on sitting in a safely installed, properly strapped car seat *every* time you are driving – even if it is down the street!

Using a proper car seat is so important. Make sure that you buy one *new* (one of the few times you really do have to buy new). A seat that has been in an accident is not safe. Car

---

312   http://www.youtube.com/watch?v=G8mFsXNXOLw

seats expire in 5 – 6 years because the plastic can break down over time – do not use an expired seat. There are safe seats in every price range, from around $50 on up to $300 or so. A convertible seat will last the longest, because it can go from newborn – 3 or 4 years (sometimes longer).

Install the seat, if possible, in the center of the back seat. Car seats should never go in the front seat, ideally, and certainly not when the air bags are enabled. An air bag inflating in an accident can kill your baby (if rear facing) or break baby's arms or legs (if forward facing). If you must have your child in the front seat, push the seat back as far as it will go and turn off the air bags.

If your car is small, you may need to choose a smaller seat to fit it. If the seat cannot be installed firmly and tightly, look for a different one that can. Radians tend to be highly rated and also narrower/fit better in smaller cars.

We personally chose to buy Britax seats – both Marathon and Roundabout. These are more expensive. They're also safer. To get a deal, look on close-out type stores that are selling brand new seats in discontinued patterns. These will be your cheapest option. Car seats can be reused for children in your family if you know they are not expired and have not been in an accident.

Cars seats also have flame retardants and other potentially toxic chemicals on them. There have been rankings of the most and least toxic seats starting in 2011[313]. Cross-reference this with safety ratings and the types of car seats that will work best for your child (size-wise) and your car to choose the best seat.

If in doubt, seek the help of a Certified Passenger Safety Technician (CPST). These people, often police or firemen but also sometimes "lay" people, can advise you on the best and safest seat for your car and child, and can help you install it properly. It is a good idea to take your seat to a free car seat check to make sure yours is installed well and that you are strapping your child in properly. Otherwise it is hard to know if your child is as safe as s/he should be in the car!

PERSONAL CARE PRODUCTS:
WHICH TO USE AND WHY

Most new parents buy mainstream brands of baby wash, baby shampoo, baby lotion, baby oil, baby powder, and more. The vast majority of these are merely marketing gimmicks, designed to get new parents to spend money on items they don't really need. Most of these also contain petroleum-based ingredients that are not very safe for baby's and children's skin!

Babies and children truly need very minimal personal care products. They really don't get very dirty, and most of the dirt they do encounter can be easily washed off with water. All the fancy, nice-smelling products (which, by the way, are scented with petroleum-derived fragrance chemicals) are just to make parents feel good, not to benefit the child. In fact, these products are poorly regulated and there is no guarantee of safety!

Choosing minimal and safe personal care products is important, because anything that is put on a child's skin (or adult's skin, for that matter) is going to absorb and get into the child's bloodstream. The skin is basically a big sponge. Therefore, a good rule is "don't put anything on your skin that you wouldn't put in your mouth." This doesn't have to be exactly literal – I wouldn't put a lotion made from plant-based oils in my mouth, although I would put the plants from which the oils came in my mouth – but the general sentiment is a good one.

A child really only needs:

- Body wash
- Shampoo or "no 'poo"
- Lotion (on occasion)

There is nothing else a child needs on a regular basis. Baby powder may be helpful in dealing with certain skin rashes, but doesn't need to be used after every change. (And when choosing a baby powder, look for one based on bentonite clay or simply use arrowroot powder.) Baby oil is petroleum oil and is not safe, nor needed. Bubble bath can prove to irritate a child's sensitive skin and may even lead to UTIs, especially in girls. These additional bath products are simply unneeded.

A basic body wash is good, but does not need to be used all the time. Good options include pure castile soap like Dr. Bronner's, or an organic/natural baby wash, like Burt's Bees. We generally use pure castile soap, either unscented or scented with essential oils only.

In many cases, a natural body wash can double as shampoo, which is fine. Burt's Bees product does, and is also tear-free. A plain castile soap is *not* tear-free. Instead, combining baking soda and water can clean hair nicely, is extremely inexpensive, very safe, and naturally tear-free. A few drops of essential oil (rosemary, bergamot, or grapefruit are good options) can be added to this mix. It really does clean hair nicely. For older girls with long hair, a homemade detangler can be made from a small amount of a plant-based oil mixed in water, and sprayed in as a leave-in option. Kids do not really need any conditioner.

Some kids deal with dry skin, especially in the winter. A healthy child who is eating plenty of saturated fats and staying hydrated shouldn't have much issue with this. However, it can happen. Newborns should not have the vernix washed off their skin (which provides both moisture and immune-boosting properties) to attempt to prevent dry skin. If a child needs a lotion, a plain plant oil, like olive, avocado, sweet almond, or grapeseed is a good idea. If a true "lotion" is desired, homemade lotions based on these plant oils are very simple to make and last a long time.

A good place to shop for other options is through WAHMs on Etsy. Most homemade options – whether by you or someone else – are fairly safe, although read the ingredients.

These products can be used on sore bottoms, dirty bottoms, sensitive skin, skin prone to eczema (which is usually a sign of an allergy), dry skin, and really any other kind. Even children who are allergic or sensitive to just about every commercial product can safely use these natural options.

A word of warning, though – avocado oil and shea butter shouldn't be used by those with latex allergies. If a child does have any food allergies, no oil associated with that food should be used on the skin. If a red rash shows up or the child has any other noticeable reaction, then the product or ingredient in question should be discontinued.

DOES YOUR CHILD *REALLY* NEED A BATH?

Many parents believe children benefit from a nightly bath. While in some ways this is true – it provides a relaxing and fun environment, as well as becoming part of a bed time routine – in other ways it is not true. Children do not *need* daily baths, anymore than adults actually do.

Bathing, especially in modern days – days of water contaminated with chloride, fluoride, and other problematic chemicals, and of harsh soaps that strip the skin's natural oils – can be more hurtful than helpful. A weekly bath is enough for most kids up until they are nearing the tween years, and then twice a week is probably enough most of the time. Infants can be bathed less often until they are mobile. New babies can wait weeks to a month before getting a first bath! (Of course, the diaper area should be cleaned gently as needed.)

Chlorine in tap water absorbs easily into the skin and isn't good for children. Some children who are bathed frequently may even suffer increased dry skin or eczema because of the water contaminants. That's just one reason to minimize baths. Water quality can be improved by a filtration system in the bathroom itself or for the whole house.

Children also do not need baths frequently to remain clean. A child can be cleaned with mostly water. They certainly don't get dirty enough on a daily basis to require a bath! Washing bottoms, hands, and faces is enough in most cases. A quick rinse in a shower is sufficient at other times.

Bathing strips the skin of its natural oils, which can cause dryness, or cause skin to overcompensate with oil production, leading to oily skin (and possibly to greasy hair or acne in tween and teen children).

We need to look at bathing as a tool to keep ourselves healthy, but not one that should be over used. Once or twice a week is sufficient; much more often is probably too much. At most a child should be rinsed off or use wash cloths to clean sticky hands, faces, and bottoms (if needed). Less bathing is more.

KEEPING HOMES ALLERGY-FREE

For parents whose children have seasonal or pet-related allergies, keeping homes clean and allergy-free is very important. Dust and dander can cause a real problem for some children.

First, see the other sections on allergies. Sometimes, these allergies are caused by underlying gut damage, and they can be helped or even reversed by the GAPS diet. Consider looking into something like this if your child is an allergy sufferer.

In the mean time, keeping the home clean and allergen-free is important. If you are dealing with food allergies, see the Food section on those, as well as the labeling tricks to help keep unsafe food out of the home.

For environmental allergies, a good air filter is helpful. A HEPA air filter can reduce allergens in the home. Consider running one in the main living space and one in the child's bedroom.

Removing carpet and replacing with tile or hardwood is a good idea. These don't trap dust the same way that carpet does, and they are easier to keep clean. A simple dust mop run over them every few days usually can keep dust and dander at bay. Carpets that do remain should be vacuumed at least weekly, more often if there is a pet in the home.

Washing curtains, towels, and bedding regularly can help keep the home allergy-free. There are certain types of pillows that are made for kids with allergies. Bedding made from natural fibers instead of synthetic will also be safer. Aim to wash bedding once a week.

Consider keeping pets outside or only allowing access to certain areas of the home (i.e. not in the child's bedroom) to keep dander down. If a child is severely allergic, the pet may need to find a new home.

Keeping mats immediately outside and inside of homes can help to keep outside "stuff" out. Shoes should be removed at the door. This is especially important if the allergies are seasonal the pollen counts are high. Look into freeze-dried nettle and raw honey to help allergy symptoms as well.

Windows should be kept closed in warm months, especially if the pollen count is high. Use the HEPA filter and replace the filter as needed, which may be more often at this time.

In general, it is not too difficult to keep homes clean and allergy-free, if a few simple precautions are taken. Continue to look into any underlying issues and consider approaching allergies from a gut/physical level if possible.

TV AND MEDIA USE IN CHILDREN

Is the TV evil?

To hear many parents tell it, it is. The TV should be avoided at all costs! Media use is making our kids fat...and stupid!

But the truth is, media use, like anything else, must have its proper place in our lives. It is a useful tool for learning and relaxation, but it must not be overused.

At this time, the average child under 13 watches about three hours of TV per day. About two-thirds of children have TVs in their bedrooms, and the average home had 4 TVs in all. Currently, this exceeds AAP guidelines, which recommend that children watch no more than two hours of TV per day[314]. The AAP also recommends that children under 2 years not watch any TV.

Children under 6 currently spend about two hours a day watching TV or using a computer[315]. This was as much as they spent playing outside, and more than they spent reading or being read to.

Free play allowed has decreased dramatically since 1970[316], and children are suffering for it. They're expecting to be "entertained" by an adult or a form of media instead of learning to play and think creatively. When TV and computers take over so much of a child's life, this is a bad thing.

Studies have also shown that TV watching can lead to poor eating habits, due to the large number of junk-food-related commercials that children view[317].

Some parents swing to the opposite extreme, never allowing their children to watch TV or use computers at all. But this, too, is a mistake. Children need to learn to "get along" with media in their lives, especially when they are older. TV, when used for the occasional educational video, is a good thing. 30 minutes per day will not hurt a child. Computers, when used for viewing or reading educational material and learning computer skills (typing, research) are also appropriate. They must be viewed as tools.

How We Handle TV and Media

Our children are allowed to watch TV. They don't have access to a TV most of the time, but there are days we watch movies because someone doesn't feel well or we're having an "off" day. We've personally found that they will only sit still for 20 – 30 minutes unless they aren't feeling well, and then they will often want to shut off the TV or ignore it in favor of more creative or hands-on activities. To them, imaginative play is usually better than TV.

We do not have live TV. We stream videos we find appropriate from the computer to the TV so that they are not exposed to commercials or anything we don't want them to watch, at this time. We don't like to watch commercials, either (and also don't watch live TV). This cuts down on the media influence.

314   http://pediatrics.aappublications.org/content/118/5/e1303.full
315   http://articles.cnn.com/2003-10-28/health/tv.kids_1_kaiser-s-vicky-rideout-study-videos?_
        s=PM:HEALTH
316   http://www.sciencedaily.com/releases/2013/01/130107110538.htm
317   http://abclocal.go.com/kabc/story?id=8217634

We choose a selection of fun kid videos. We like the KidsTV123 channel on Youtube. We choose "How It's Made" videos. We watch Thomas the Train, Bob the Builder, and Duck Tales a lot. Shaun the Sheep is another favorite. Super Book, a very old Bible-based cartoon, is something else they watch. We tend *not* to choose fast moving, flashy cartoons or anything one might find on Nickelodeon or The Disney Channel.

Finally, they only use computers very minimally, perhaps less than 30 minutes per week. We don't feel they need to at their ages (our oldest is 5). We will occasionally let them sit with us and type or play a game, but this is very rare. When they are older and can read, they will learn to use computers at that point.

TV and computers aren't evil. They won't ruin children. Poor use and overuse have a negative impact on children – watching several hours per day, watching TV instead of playing imaginatively and learning to think creatively, being exposed to lots of fast-moving shows and commercials. TV in small doses, as a tool for occasional relaxation, learning, and so on is fine.

All parents choose to handle TV a bit differently. Some allow their children unrestricted access (and we have done this at different points) because their children often will ignore the TV in favor of other activities anyway. Some are strict about a 30-minutes-per-day rule because their children will simply sit and watch as long as it is on. It is up to each parent to know their child and make rules that fit their family best.

POSITIVE DISCIPLINE METHODS

These days, there's a real push towards a punitive model of discipline. Many parents believe that "kids today" are spoiled, self-centered, and need more discipline in order to turn out as decent citizens. More are spanking, and some have turned to public humiliation as a means of getting through to a child. These methods are often celebrated by parents, who believe that without punishment, a child can't learn to behave.

This is false, and a complete misunderstanding of developmental psychology. Children learn to behave by observing the behavior of those around them and mimicking what they see. They also go through normal developmental stages – including biting, hitting, toy-stealing, selfishness, and so on. No amount of punishment can prevent them from going through these stages or make them get past these stages faster. Parents who believe they can simply punish their children and "they will know better" do not understand this.

That is not to say that children shouldn't have boundaries and consequences – they should. As much as possible consequences should be naturally imposed. Boundaries should be centered around having respect for other people and property. A child may not hit someone else, take their toy, push or poke, or deliberately break an object.

The ultimate goal in parenting is to stop any behaviors or actions that break these boundaries. Punishment is not the only way to stop them, or even the most desirable way to stop them. Especially for young children, exploring the underlying cause of the behavior is more effective than simply punishing them. When parents can keep in mind that their goal is to *stop the behavior*, and not to *punish the child*, and they can separate these two ideas, they can maintain a more positive and peaceful home.

For example, if a 3 or 4-year-old begins the behavior of shoving a baby or young toddler sibling randomly (i.e. not provoked by the younger child taking a toy or 'doing something' to cause), most parents will be horrified, desire to protect the younger child, and want to punish the older child for hurting the younger. "They must learn this is not acceptable! They must not hurt the smaller child!" And this is true – the pushing behavior needs to stop, in order to protect the younger child's safety and bodily integrity. But what is most effectively going to accomplish that goal?

Punishment may or may not work. In cases like this, the driving motivation is often jealousy towards the younger child and a feeling of disconnect from the parents, a desire for attention. If the child gets attention – even negative attention – for pushing the child (plus it "soothes" their anger and jealousy to act out towards the other child), then they will actually keep doing it. This is counterproductive to the ultimate goal!

Instead, if a parent pulls the older child close and says, "Are you feeling sad? Do you need a hug?" and holds onto them, something entirely different happens. This is counterintuitive to what we have been taught that "naughty children deserve," but think about this. After hugging the child, the parent should quietly say, "You may not hurt your sibling. If you are feeling sad, come and ask me for a hug." The child, having received the positive attention needed and feeling soothed and connected, as well as having been told what to do instead, will come and seek a hug instead of pushing. I used this method on one of my own children and the pushing behavior was a very, very short phase after that. Punishment did not work; connecting did.

A positive parent looks for ways to keep boundaries firm and keep everyone safe, while accepting everyone's feelings and helping them to express those feelings in a more appropriate way. We might say "It's not okay to call your brother a stupid-head; you may say 'I don't like it when you push me.'" We give the children words to use instead of the ones we find inappropriate. We give them the words to use instead of actions. "It's not okay to push your sister; you may say 'Excuse me, please move.'"

Children learn their behavior from an example of what *to* do, and not through being punished for wrong actions. They need to be held accountable and they need the boundaries to be firm, but they do not need to be punished. Natural consequences are important.

For example, if a child hits another child and that child begins to cry, they have to deal with having hurt a friend and needing to make that friend feel better. They should be encouraged to do so – "Look, she seems sad. Can you help her feel better?" Many children will spontaneously apologize at this point. (And a child too young or too frustrated to arrive at that conclusion might be gently prompted – but not forced – to apologize. Continued poor behavior should result in the end of the play date so that the child's underlying need, perhaps food, sleep, or just a break, can be met.)

At no time is a child's poor behavior *ignored*. At no time is their poor behavior *excused*. Parents do not say "Oh, she's just being spirited! Let her have the toy." If a toy is taken, it is gently removed from the child's hands and given back to the original child, as the parent gently says "It is her turn right now. You may have a turn when she is done." Then the child is removed to another part of the room and given something else to do. The child is not punished – but the child does not get to keep the toy she stole.

Thinking this way about parenting is radically different, and may not make sense to everyone. That's okay. Every parent and every child are different, and the method of "handling" a child or situation will vary. Nobody has all the answers. Also, this book isn't primarily about discipline; it's mentioned here only briefly. There are many great resources out there for those who are interested in learning more about this idea. It is helpful to be surrounded by people who believe the same way and who can serve as a support, especially for someone who is new to the idea.

Even for parents who choose to approach parenting differently, trying to meet a child's needs and maintain a positive environment when possible will benefit everyone.

SCHOOLING OPTIONS

Every parent comes to a point where they must consider schooling for their children. All children require an education of some sort. While public school has been the typical option for the last 50 years or so, it's no longer the only option. Many parents are opting for private or charter schools, or are choosing to home school. There are even a variety of methods of home schooling out there.

Each family is different, and each child is different. Every child's needs will be best served in a slightly different setting. The child's individual needs must be balanced with the family's situation and needs (for example: are there multiple siblings? Do any have special needs? Do both parents work? What type of school setting do the parents desire for their family?).

Schooling can be a huge decision and a huge discussion, but we will look at a quick overview of the options here.

Public School

Unfortunately, public schools vary widely by district, and even within districts. They can be excellent, or not so much. Choosing "public school" is therefore dependent on what is available in your area. Many classrooms have between 15 and 40 children (averaging 25 – 30) and are obviously grouped by grade level. Excellent schools have remedial programs available to help students who need extra help and have parent volunteers come in to work with them as well. Excellent schools also offer special gifted programs, and extra-curricular activities on a wide range of topics.

Less excellent schools often have a higher teacher-to-student ratio, less help for students who are struggling or exceptional, less parent involvement, and fewer extra-curricular activities. Investigate the schools in your area carefully to see how they are. Public school may be a good or bad thing, depending on the child, family, and how good the school is.

Private School

Private schools also vary. They can be very expensive, which is cost-prohibitive for some families. They often have smaller classes, from 10 – 20 students, and more individualized attention. But they are not all the same. There are private schools that focus on different subjects ("arts" schools, "science and math" schools, etc.). There are also private schools that focus on entirely different educational philosophies – Waldorf, Montessori, etc.

A private school may be a good place for a child who, whether due to learning style, learning disabilities, or giftedness, needs a more individualized education. If parents can afford it and desire to send their children to a school, a private option can allow for a better 'fit' for the child than whatever school district they are in – although it depends on the school district and the private options.

One drawback is that private schools are often small and may not have the same depth of extra-curricular activities that public schools do. Also, tuition can be a couple thousand to several thousand dollars per year.

Homeschooling

For some parents, the best education happens at home. Home school can be entirely tailored to each student, because the parent is only dealing with a small number of children, whom they know well. A wide variety of educational philosophies can be used, depending on the parent/child. A child is capable of moving at his/her own pace with the different subjects, possibly jumping ahead in some and going slower with others. The sheer individual nature makes homeschooling ideal for many children.

However, home schooling requires a lot of work and sacrifice on the part of the parents. In most cases, the parent needs to be home with the children all day – so both parents can't work full-time. The parent also needs to seek out appropriate curriculum or create their own, which can be overwhelming to some. The parent also is the sole person motivating the child to learn, rather than having a "neutral" teacher involved – and this can be a battle in some cases.

These days, there are lots of home school groups and activities so that parents can receive support and help, and children can learn from other parents and socialize with other kids. Some public schools allow home schooled kids to play sports or participate in other activities.

The families that choose to home school usually feel very passionately about it and really enjoy it. Others find the amount of time and sacrifice required overwhelming, or are unable to quit work or arrange their schedule so they can be there to do it, even if they would like to.

Parents who are intrigued by home schooling but who don't or can't commit to doing it can send their children to school and supplement with activities at home as desired.

The Bottom Line

There is far more to the schooling debate than this; this is a *very* brief overview. Each family must thoroughly consider what is right for them.

If possible, talk to families who have made different choices in education to get a feel for what each is really like. There are a lot of pre-conceived notions about each option that may be faulty (such as public school is just for drones, or home schooled kids don't socialize). Read about different options and methods. Visit the schools in your area and talk to the teachers, staff, and families who attend there. Get a feel for what's available. Choose what works best for your family.

We have chosen to home school for a wide variety of reasons, but that is what works for us. Every family will be different.

CLOSING

This book was quite the undertaking – it has over 300 sources and took me a couple hundred hours to put together. It was fascinating to write and research and I hope it's been helpful to you. Feel free to flip through it, bookmark the parts you liked or found important, and to reference it often.

There were *so* many questions and topics and so much feedback that I got from my readers and editors throughout the process of writing this book that it was literally impossible to include everything. This book is merely an overview, a tiny bit of insight into some major child-rearing issues. It can't cover everything and it's not an exhaustive resource. See my Resources section for additional books to read on topics that interest you.

In the future I may write additional books to answer additional questions in these areas, or to look at different age groups. There's not a lot in here on babies or pregnancy because that was simply a huge topic in and of itself! Someday, perhaps!

Thanks for reading!

A Practical Guide to Children's Health